Recovery from Illness

ology for Fitness

WILEY SERIES ON
DEVELOPMENTS IN NURSING RESEARCH
VOLUME I

Recovery from Illness

JENIFER WILSON-BARNETT, B.A., M.Sc., Ph.D., S.R.N., Dip.N., R.N.T.
and
MORVA FORDHAM, B.Sc., M.Sc., S.R.N., S.C.M., R.N.T.
Department of Nursing Studies
Chelsea College
University of London

with contributions by

LYNN BATEHUP, S.R.N., Dip.N.
St. George's Hospital
London, and Chelsea College, University of London

CECILY PARTRIDGE, B.A., F.C.S.P.
Chelsea College
University of London

CHRISTINE WEBB, B.A., M.Sc., S.R.N., R.S.C.N., R.N.T.
Chelsea College
University of London

A Wiley Medical Publication

175 YEARS OF PUBLISHING
1807 1982

JOHN WILEY & SONS
Chichester · New York · Brisbane · Toronto · Singapore

Library of Congress Cataloging in Publication Data:

Wilson-Barnett, Jenifer.
Recovery from illness.
(A Wiley medical publication)
Bibliography: p.
Includes index.
1. Postoperative care. 2. Convalescence.
3. Rehabilitation nursing. I. Fordham, Morva.
II. Title. III. Series.
RD51.W54 616 82-2739

ISBN 0 471 10408 6 AACR2

British Library Cataloguing in Publication Data:

Wilson-Barnett, Jenifer
Recovery from illness. — (Wiley series in development and nursing research; vol. 1)
1. Sick — Psychology
I. Title II. Fordham, Morva
616 R726.5

ISBN 0 471 10408 6

Phototypeset by Dobbie Typesetting Service, Plymouth, Devon and printed by Pitman Press Ltd., Bath, Avon.

Contents

Series Preface

Developments in Nursing Research

Nursing science is derived from an integration of knowledge in other disciplines and from original nursing research studies. As more relevant research is completed key areas are developing, benefitting from different approaches in various patient care settings. The purpose of this series is to publish literature reviews and original material in such areas to promote nursing progress and knowledge.

Introduction

This book aims to review the research evidence on aspects of patients' recovery from illness, and to present studies in this area. By 'recovery' we mean the process of returning to the patient's pre-morbid level of health. For a few this may be too optimistic, but certainly for the majority of patients recovering from acute episodes or surgery this should be total. The usage of the term is therefore quite specific and differs from 'rehabilitation', which commonly infers a long-term process of adjustment to permanent incapacity. The time span, or the types of illness and the staff involved, are therefore different.

Physical illness can arise in many different ways. It can strike the previously healthy as well as the chronically sick and the disabled. The routes to recovery may be tortuous and diverse, but it is crucial that the patient and the health-care personnel agree the ultimate goal and the criteria used to judge its attainment.

Recovery is a process whereby a person moves from a state of illness to a state of health. One dictionary (*Dorland*, 1965) defines illness as 'a condition marked by pronounced deviation from the normal state of health'. The World Health Organization has defined health as 'a state of complete physical, mental and social well-being and not merely the absence of disease or infirmity'. These broad definitions containing evaluative words such as 'pronounced deviation' and 'well-being' are open to interpretation. Different groups of people use differing criteria against which to measure illness and health.

Recovery from illness is often a cooperative venture involving any number of participants—family, friends, employers, medical and para-medical personnel and society at large—all of whom may have differing views of health and illness. As the aim of the exercise is to enable and assist the ill person regain health, the views of illness and health taken by the patient are of central importance (with the possible exception of the newborn and the mentally ill). When does an individual regard himself as ill and seek health care? Statisticians (White *et al.*, 1961) have emphasized that only a minority of persons who are ill enter the health-care system; this proportion was estimated to be about one-third. A multitude of physical and psychological factors influence the individual's view of his state of health and his entry into the health-care system (Kohn and Kerr, 1976). However, multivariate analysis (White *et al.*, 1967; White and Murnaghan, 1969) revealed that illness for the majority of patients was characterized by restriction of activity and discomfort. Illness from the sick person's point of view, or 'patient-perceived morbidity', was defined by restricted activity and discomforting symptoms. The goal of recovery from illness from the patient's perspective is the resumption of habitual activity and the absence of discomfort. However, the medical definition of physical illness or 'clinical morbidity' is not generally described by the behaviour and subjective feelings of the sick, but primarily in terms of abnormality of structure and function of the body. The physician's role is customarily that of investigating, diagnosing and treating biological and psychological dysfunction. Patient-perceived morbidity may or may not correspond with clinical morbidity, but the two are generally regarded as correlated but conceptually distinct variables. Problems for recovery from illness arise when these concepts are not correlated, if the patient regards himself as healthy despite abnormal clinical signs, or if the patient feels ill and clinical evidence cannot be found. Such circumstances result in a mismatch of goals and much conflict, resolved either by separation of the two parties or by acceptance of the other person's point of view and goals.

Clinical morbidity	*Patient-perceived morbidity*
Biological or psychological dysfunction	Restricted activity and discomfort

		Clinical morbidity YES	Clinical morbidity NO
Patient-perceived morbidity	YES	I	III
	NO	II	IV

Figure 1

Figure 1 illustrates the relationship between clinical and patient-perceived morbidity. The person with chronic disease aims to move from Group I to Group II, or at least to a position where perceived morbidity is less than during the acute illness. The cooperative venture of hospice care has demonstrated the extent to which patient goals (activity and comfort) can be achieved even when clinical morbidity cannot be overcome.

The erstwhile healthy person suffering acute illness is presumed to transfer from Group I to Group IV; however, many patients linger in Group III, attributing continued discomfort and inability to resume normal activities to illness that occurred weeks, months, or years before. Contact between patients and health carers is generally close and continuous only during the acute stages of illness, and both tend to assume that when clinical goals have been achieved patient goals will automatically follow. Even when patient and health carer achieve mutual understanding and agreement on goals, they are likely to use different criteria for judging recovery. Each group uses the criteria which they are in the best position to judge. Medical criteria are predominantly related to bodily structure and function, are objective and based upon statistically determined ranges of normality. Patients criteria are predominantly related to their lifestyle, are subjective and based upon idiosyncratic values. The dichotomy is obviously not absolute. The ill person can observe signs himself (e.g. external bleeding, wound state) and health carers can indirectly observe symptoms (e.g. pain and fatigue).

An important aim of research on recovery is to elucidate the relationship between objective and subjective criteria. It is recognized that the patient's perception of 'shortness of breath' is not correlated 100% with objective lung function (Hale *et al.*, 1977), nor does a patient's report of the quality of sleep correspond with objective recordings of sleep EEG's (Kavey and Altshiler, 1979).

A second aim of recovery research is to investigate the application of positive criteria of health such as physical fitness and to develop patient advice regarding behaviour which will hasten recovery.

The need for work in this area is indicated by the growing evidence that technical success from surgery is not enough to restore patients to their optimum state of health. For those who undergo elective surgery, a complete cure is usually expected. However, patient and surgeon may have different expectations during recovery, and their perceptions of when optimum recovery has been achieved sometimes vary. This often leads to problems for patients in the short and long term, but on return home they often assume that they are well once discharged and are quite shocked by their degree of weakness and tiredness, whereas staff are not at all surprised! However, one thing that constantly interests surgeons is the variability in speed of recovery and how quickly some patients become active and independent while others require assistance and sometimes further treatment for what appears to be the same degree of the same disorder. This may be accounted for by several social, psychological and physical parameters.

Many areas of post-operative care, which might influence recovery, could be improved. These must be demonstrated by research and scientific principles. We have been hindered too long by trial and error and individualistic approaches and need far more knowledge about the contributory factors. This book represents an attempt to highlight some of the gaps in knowledge and to explore other areas to provide more information and explanation.

Most of the valuable research in following up patients after surgery, evaluating morbidity and complications reviewed in this book, is undertaken by doctors. However, the subject of recovery is also of great relevance to others. It could, for instance, be described as of central importance to nurses and physiotherapists.

This book addresses itself to such questions as:

What factors affect the speed of recovery?
How can 'recovery' be measured?
Are there any useful maxims to suggest an optimum level of activity throughout recovery?
Are certain patients 'at risk' of a poor post-operative recovery?
What intervention can be indicated to prevent delayed recovery?

Apart from reviewing our current level of knowledge, several original studies are presented at length. They each offer a different approach and research methods and study specific groups of patients. Fordham's research draws on physiological and ergonomic principles, assessing male herniorrhaphy patients' perceptions of their fitness in relation to physical measurement of fitness, their experiences and activities during the immediate post-operative period and after their return to work. In contrast, Wilson-Barnett's studies emphasize the psychological factors that influence recovery. The follow-up study with cardiac patients aims to correlate psychological dimensions with patients' reports of their physical status and experiences during the post-operative year. Other surgery which causes mutilation or affects patients' self-perception is also reviewed. Much of this research demonstrates that personality factors are important determinants but that specific interventions can reduce some unnecessary morbidity.

The next section by Lynn Batehup, discussing the early care of stroke patients, demonstrates how prevention of permanent spasticity may result from correct early application of the Bobath principles. This involves patients frequently discussed in texts on rehabilitation because of their protracted need for care and treatment. It demonstrates that nurses should accept their positive contribution for this large group of patients, after which much of the recovery process is aided by the individual's effort to function with the aid of physiotherapy and, where necessary, speech therapy. This longer-term process is discussed by a leading physiotherapist, Cecily Partridge, analysing the relationships between 'impairment' and 'handicap'.

Finally, methods to prevent unnecessary morbidity after surgery and illness are reviewed in a positive attempt to draw from research some guidelines for practice. The whole subject has immense implications for patient care, the dynamics of nursing and medicine, and of course for avoiding further financial burden for the NHS. Perhaps in a small way this book may motivate more thought on longer-term recovery and some interventions which avoid unnecessary distress for patients.

References

Dorland's Illustrated Medical Dictionary (1965). W. B. Saunders Co., Philadelphia and London.

Hale, T., Spuggs, J., and Hamley, E. J. (1977). The effects of an exercise regime on patients with living malfunction. *British Journal of Sports Medicine*, **11**, 181.

Kavey, N. B., and Altshiler, K. Z. (1979). Sleep in herniorrhaphy patients. *American Journal of Surgery*, **138**, 682–687.

Kohn, R., and Kerr, L. W. (Editors) (1976). *Health Care: An International Study*. Oxford University Press, London.

White, K. L., and Murnaghan, J. H. (1969). International comparisons of medical care utilization—a feasibility study. *National Centre for Health Statistics, Public Health Service Publication No. 1000*, Series 2, No. 33. US Government Printing Office, Washington, DC.

White, K. L., Williams, T. F., and Greenberg, B. G. (1961). The ecology of medical care. *New England Journal of Medicine*, **265**, 885–892.

White, K. L., Andjelkovic, D., Pearson, R. J. C., Mabry, J. H., Ross, A., and Sogan, O. K. (1967). International comparisons of medical care utilization. *New England Journal of Medicine*, **277**, 516–522.

CHAPTER 1

Rest, Inactivity, and Sleep during Recovery

'The treatment was successful but the patient still felt ill.'

The blood picture is normal, the wound has healed, yet the patient still complains of constipation, anorexia, weakness, aches and apathy. How often do we encounter this situation during the recovery period? How many people attribute fatigue and failure to enjoy life to the full to an illness, injury or operation that occurred weeks, months, or even years before?

There are a number of well-recognized risk factors associated with delayed recovery, illustrated in Figure 2, which include age, obesity, undernutrition, tobacco consumption, underlying chronic disease, lack of fitness, and added physical or psychosocial stress.

Obesity not only increases the risks associated with operation and anaesthesia but also imposes problems during rehabilitation, especially following injury or stroke. Undernutrition can reduce muscle strength as was demonstrated by Keys *et al.* in 1950. After 12 weeks on a diet of 1570 calories per day, healthy subjects were found to have a 20% reduction in handgrip and backlift strength. Undernutrition has manifold consequences other than diminished muscle mass—reduced immunity, susceptibility to infection and poor wound healing among them. Jung's (1981) review of malnutrition in hospital makes sobering reading. The malnutrition of cancer patients and those suffering from liver diseases are important and well-recognized, but what was less expected and more easily dealt with was the malnutrition of the general medical and surgical patient.

The percentage of patients in America and Britain with malnutrition on admission to hospital varies between diagnostic groups. Bollet and Owen (1973) reported that 64% of those with alcoholic liver disease, over 30% of those with chronic obstructive airways disease and rheumatoid

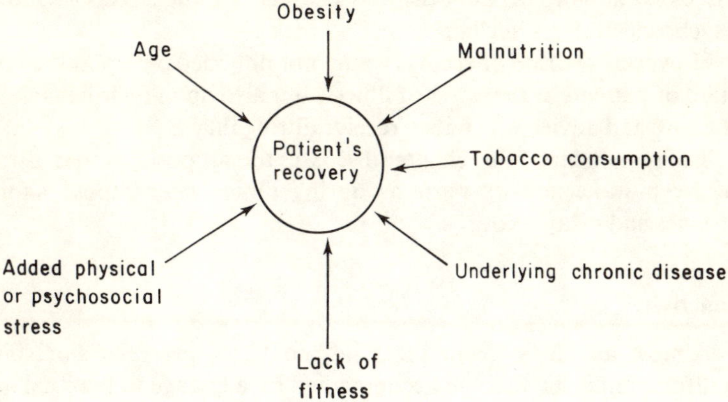

Figure 2 Risk factors

arthritis, 20% of those with peptic ulcers, 13% of those with cardiovascular disease, but only 7% of patients with diabetes mellitus had a reduced protein status. A study in Leeds (Hill *et al.*, 1977) found that 20% of those admitted for minor surgery and 40% for major surgery were malnourished, but worse than that was the finding that the prevalence of malnutrition increased during hospitalization, reaching 55% at one week after major surgery. Almost every surgical patient and many patients undergoing investigations with or without anaesthesia are required to fast. Others fail to eat in sufficient quantity (Hackett *et al.*, 1979). Control over the nutrition of patients is a shared responsibility which, for different patients and at differing stages of their illness, may be taken primarily by doctors, dieticians or nurses. The concerted effort of all concerned is necessary to ensure optimal nutrition.

Tobacco consumption not only increases anaesthetic risk and the incidence of post-operative respiratory complications, but it is also associated with chronic cardiovascular and respiratory pathology. Bradshaw (1981), in a discussion on the assessment of patients prior to operation and anaesthesia, suggests that, in addition to medical history and physical examination, a simple exercise tolerance test to such activities as climbing stairs may be desirable, since it was established by Kyei-Mensah and Thornton (1974) that between 26 and 40% of surgical patients have underlying medical diseases—particularly cardiorespiratory problems. The sophistication and skill of modern anaesthesia and operating techniques makes it possible for any patient to undergo anaesthesia. The relationship between physical fitness and recovery is discussed in more detail in the next chapter and the effects of additional psychosocial stress in Chapter 3.

However, the rate of recovery may not only depend upon the physical state of patients at the onset of illness, but also upon their behaviour and the care and advice which they receive during illness.

The remainder of this chapter discusses the proposition that disruption of sleep–wake–activity patterns during illness may impose additional stresses and delay recovery.

Inactivity

Almost all illness from the mild 'cold' to severe cardiorespiratory malfunction is likely to be accompanied by a change in habitual activity patterns. The proposition that patients regard themselves as ill and in need of care when sickness curtails their ability to remain normally active was discussed briefly in the Introduction.

Why does a sick person curtail his activities? Considering the integration of body systems demanded by muscular work it is small wonder that illness for the majority of patients is characterized by difficulty in maintaining normal activities. There is no one explanation of the change in behaviour. In some instances injury or infection interferes with the transfer of oxygen from air to muscles; some illnesses affect neuromuscular activity. When pain is exacerbated by movement it will be avoided. Physical illness may be the culmination of stress (Sterling and Eyer, 1981), and withdrawal from the 'daily round' may be psychologically motivated and advocated. However, inactivity resulting from illness may be compounded by treatment. The sedative effects of analgesic, antihistaminic, antiemetic and hypnotic drugs further increase the sick person's desire to be inactive (Weber *et al.*, 1975), as do the effects of anaesthesia and operation. The attitude of health professionals and the environment in which the sick person is placed generally reinforce the association of illness with inactivity. The wearing of 'night-clothes', the lack of space and suitable places to walk, and the desire of staff to account for the whereabouts of patients at all times impose subtle and unsubtle pressure on patients to limit activity.

Rest

The fashion for bedrest has passed its heyday. In a seminal book, John Hilton wrote in 1878 about the value of rest as an aid to nature's healing process. He proposed that systems of the body—alimentary, cardiovascular, etc.—could be rested just as effectively as the surgeon rested a broken bone or a large wound. Browse (1965) in *The Physiology and Pathology of Bedrest* suggested that misinterpretation of this thesis led physicians to go 'overboard' for rest to cure every ill, and that in the mid-19th century the bed had become the 'king' of medicine. Asher's (1947) graphic description of the patient lying long in bed—'the blood clotting in his veins, the lime draining from his bones, the scybala stacking up in his colon, the flesh rotting from his seat, the urine leaking from his distended bladder and the spirit evaporating from his soul'—did much to topple the bed from its throne. Most patients today are out of bed within a day or two of surgery and the length of bedrest prescribed for medical conditions is diminishing. Yet patients rarely feel strong or energetic following illness. Two explanations for this state of affairs are generally given: one that the feeling of fatigue is the response to the stress of illness, the other that the patient has become unfit as a result of inactivity.

Fatigue

The word fatigue is in common parlance and seems intuitively valid, yet it is extremely difficult to describe or measure in objective terms. Historically the main thrust of research on fatigue has not been related to illness but to industrial productivity. Indeed, the Industrial Health Research Board was originally called the Industrial Fatigue Research Board. Signs of fatigue in systems of the body can be elicited. When the physical stress of particular work is investigated, physiological signs of strain can be measured (Brouha, 1960). Monitoring of physiological parameters such as temperature, pulse, blood pressure and blood lactate are used to note if and how long it takes for a return to resting values. This type of investigation has proved helpful in deciding whether an individual is able to cope with physical work without developing cumulative fatigue over hours, days, or weeks. As other forms of energy superseded that generated by human muscles and technology changed the nature of work, the concept was related to psychological factors such as vigilance and motivation (Bartlett, 1953). From time to time those who have reviewed the research on fatigue (Cameron, 1973) have concluded that it is a redundant concept—a generalized response to stress over a period of time, or so multifaceted as to be less than useful. However, intervention that reduces stress (Wilson-Barnett, 1979) may reduce subjective fatigue.

Muscle fatigue, the failure to generate or maintain force, is a less-ambiguous concept and may arise from failure in any part of the command chain—brain, spinal cord, peripheral nerve, neuromuscular junction, or muscle. Fatigue of individual muscles or groups of muscles is liable to occur when strength has been lost by underuse or when muscles not designed for the task are required to maintain posture or produce movement.

Maintaining an upright posture for standing and walking becomes more fatiguing when curvature and flexure of the neck, spine or knees—provoked by continual sitting in bed or chair—force muscles unaccustomed and not designed for the task to keep the centre of gravity over the feet. This can be a particular problem for the elderly as the strength of back muscles drops faster with age than of muscles of the hands and arms (Simonson, 1947; Aniansson, 1978). It is important that strength is not further reduced during illness. There is a diurnal variation of strength, with less strength in the early morning rising during the morning, the exact pattern depending upon the sleep-wake pattern of the individual. Jeanneret and Webb (1963), for instance, recorded a 13% variation in handgrip between early morning and afternoon.

When illness or injury specifically involves neuromusculoskeletal integrity, exercises to improve strength are administered by physio- and occupational therapists. However, loss of strength due to inactivity is liable to affect all patients to some extent. Explanation and encouragement of active muscle contraction during recovery could help all patients regain their strength more quickly.

Increase in strength with training can be considerable. On the whole, the lower the initial strength the greater the increase that can occur with training. Hettinger (1961) found that the greatest improvement in the strength of any muscle group could be obtained with a single maximum isometric muscle contraction against a resistance held for only 1–2 seconds a day. There was no additional increase in strength with more than a single contraction per day. However, improvement in strength can be achieved by contractions of only 40–50% of maximum provided the duration is increased; 60% of maximum had to be maintained for 4–6 seconds once daily to achieve the same training effect as a maximum effort held for 1–2 seconds. When the strongest daily muscle contraction fell below 20% of the maximum, regardless of the duration, then strength decreased. When 20–30% maximum muscle strength was used, strength remained stable. This, Hettinger suggests, is the range of normal daily activity where repetition of the same effort produced neither an increase nor a decrease in strength. When no tension is exerted throughout the day, loss of strength occurs at the rate of approximately 3% per day (Kottke, 1966).

Inactivity not only reduces strength but also affects the flexibility of joints and the efficiency of neuromuscular coordination necessary for skilled movement.

Flexibility of Joints

> 'Impairment of mobility due to shortening or fixation of connective tissue aggravates the problem of impairment of muscular strength and endurance.' (Kottke, 1966).

If a joint is immobilized dense connective tissue is laid down and can cause restriction of motion. This will occur in less than a week of immobilization and if, in addition to immobility, trauma or impaired circulation exists, additional collagen fibres will be laid down in as short a time as three days. According to Kottke, clinical experience suggests that joints of the lower extremities, especially the hip, which have strong muscles and heavy connective tissue, are particularly difficult to remobilize once contractures have occurred. The problems and avoiding action are most obvious for orthopaedic, rheumatic and paralysed patients (see Chapter 6). It is possible that some degree of limitation of movement occurs in the less-dramatic situation where, because of acute illness or operation, a patient is confined to bed in a semirecumbent or sitting posture, and if transferred to a chair does so without ever fully extending, let alone hyperextending, the hip, knee, lumbar and cervical joints. How often does a patient lie completely pillowless, supine or prone, or stand and walk in a fully upright posture? Kottke advocates actively or, if necessary, passively moving all joints through their full range of movement twice daily to avoid loss of flexibility.

Kelly (1966) described 'Range of Motion Exercises' for all bedfast patients. The aim is not rehabilitation but prevention of stiffness. These exercises can be performed lying supine in bed with patients who are neither paralysed nor staying in bed for many days, and once taught many patients can continue them without supervision. Kelly stressed that movement of ankles, knees, hips and spine are particularly important as normal standing posture is not being maintained during bedrest.

Skill

Skill is a sensorimotor activity in which the coordination and sequencing of neuromuscular activity are nicely adapted to the task in hand. Skills are developed par excellence in the virtuoso athlete, musician or typist, but much more humble activities like rising from a chair, dressing, and climbing stairs are skilled, and as such require practice to become and remain perfect. When illness or injury primarily affects neuromuscular function resulting in loss of skill, the patient learns or relearns under the tuition of a physio-, occupational, or speech therapist, or remedial gymnast.

Reinforcement of that learning by nurses is necessary to ensure that the patient performs tasks in the manner in which he has been taught. However, reduction in strength, endurance and flexibility may force patients in much less obvious circumstances to perform particular tasks in new ways—in effect, learning a new skill or adapting an old one. Close observation and careful questioning may reveal all manner of activities that patients have adapted on their own initiative—walking, climbing stairs, lifting, getting in and out of bed, sexual intercourse. It is emerging from current research (Fordham, Webb, Gould, and Wilson-Barnett) that various groups of surgical patients spend much time and thought agonizing about the solution to these very questions. Relatively unsupervized convalescence can lead patients to presume that such habitual activities are trivial in the eyes of the medical and paramedical staff. The livelihood of professional athletes and musicians so obviously depends upon their skill that specialized advice is sought and given following illness or injury. Sapega and Nicholas (1981) describe the detailed assessment considered vital in the evaluation and rehabilitation of athletes. Profile data including biographical information, anthropometry, flexibility of joints and muscle strength, endurance and power output are obtained during health. These data are used to identify significant abnormalities—usually thought to be a result of returning to competition before full rehabilitation. Competitive athletes are not considered fully rehabilitated until they 'regain their own normal musculoskeletal characteristics and capabilities'. The livelihood of many more people depends upon their ability to climb stairs and lift, and a feeling of well-being may be engendered by modest skill in social recreational activities like dancing and sports. A systematic assessment of the strength, skill and habitual activities of all medical and surgical patients would enable us to advise on remedial exercises, and set positive goals for recovery.

Rest and Activity

A major dilemma for the sick and for those who care for and advise them is when to rest and when to be active. When does muscular activity interfere with the healing process, and when does rest reduce physical fitness and prolong the feeling of malaise? Kottke (1966) argues that 'function increases with use' and 'what we don't use we lose'. For any organ, functional capacity is less than the maximal physiological potential and it is developed and maintained by the usual rate of metabolic activity. 'If the rate of metabolic activity of an organ is increased, the functional capacity increases, whereas rest or inactivity results in a decrease in functional capacity. If an organ is injured, the functional capacity is reduced. If the pathological damage is permanent, the maximum physiological potential is reduced permanently. If, after injury, the metabolic activity imposed on that organ exceeds the functional capacity, exhaustion occurs and functional capacity is decreased further. At that time rest restricts activity within the capacity of the organ, so that recovery can occur, and following recovery functional capacity may increase again. Properly selected activity at that time will increase functional capacity, whereas prolonged inactivity will cause a further decrease in functional capacity.' (Kottke (1966).

It follows from this argument that during the acute stage of illness the organ or system of the body affected should be rested. When clinical signs of illness have diminished or disappeared, graduated activity should be instituted until the activity is fully restored. The same theory and practice applies to a broken limb or a handled gut. However, organs and systems of the body do not function in isolation and many decisions concern the desirability or otherwise of *total* body rest during acute illness and the amount of activity or exercise to be taken during recovery.

The integration and interdependence of all organs and systems of the body pose a great practical problem if rest of some part and activity of the remainder are desirable. Kottke's argument when applied to the whole body is in effect discussing physical fitness. The World Health Organization has defined fitness as 'the ability to perform muscular work satisfactorily'. Muscular work makes demands on almost all systems of the body. Shephard (1969) summarized these demands when describing physical fitness as follows:

> 'In an effort of brief duration (less than one minute) physical fitness depends to a large extent upon muscle strength, coordination, agility, motivation and the rate and extent of development of an oxygen debt in the active tissue. In activity of moderate duration (one minute to one hour) physical fitness is still influenced by all of the above factors, but they become progressively subordinate to the ability to transfer oxygen from the atmosphere to the working

> muscles. In protracted activity (longer than one hour) there is again a change of emphasis. Physical fitness becomes increasingly dependent on the extent and availability of the food reserves in the active tissue, and the capacity to replenish these reserves either from diet or from depots elsewhere within the body. The capacity to dissipate body heat and the establishment of an appropriate balance between the intake of water and its loss in sweat and exhaled gas also assume increasing importance.'

Illness may adversely affect any of these processes but, provided that the level of demands remains within functional limits, many patients can remain active during illness. Physical fitness is discussed in more detail in the next chapter; suffice it to say that stagnation of blood, lymph and gastrointestinal contents may predispose the patient to other general complaints such as anorexia, constipation and apathy. Activity would improve all more surely than piecemeal treatment of each symptom.

The level of activity is not the only aspect of life that changes during illness. The pattern of sleep is also likely to change, particularly when patients are admitted to hospital.

Sleep

The majority of sleep research has been performed on healthy subjects. The physiological functioning of the brain, muscles and cardiac and respiratory systems during sleep have been recorded, as well as the effects of total and selective sleep deprivation on performance, behaviour and subsequent sleep. Reviews of this research can be found in Colquhoun (1971, 1972) and Minors and Waterhouse (1981). The effect of stimulants and hypnotics on sleep have been well documented (Hartmann, 1978; Jestico, 1980). Drug manufacturers have expended a major effort in the search for a drug that will promote sleep without also disrupting the pattern of sleep cycles.

The relationship between sleep and illness is complex. Lack of sleep may precede or predispose a person to succumb to illness. Characteristic patterns of sleep accompany depressed or anxious states. Discomfort of body or mind may deprive a person of sleep. Research into the interrelationships of sleep, illness and ageing go on apace, although a consensus of opinion has yet to be achieved (Butler, 1979).

Sleep is regarded by health professions and the sick alike as essential for recovery from illness. Paradoxically, research indicates that medical, surgical and nursing intervention can all cause sleep deprivation.

The philosophical debate as to why or whether sleep is necessary goes on. Sleep research has attempted to answer two questions relevant to recovery. Firstly, what happens during sleep? The theory that brain restitution occurs during REM (rapid eye movements) sleep and body restitution during non-REM sleep has been challenged by Horne (1980). He argues that the peak in human growth hormone found during non-REM sleep (Takahashi *et al.*, 1968) may not facilitate optimal protein synthesis and mitosis since nutrient levels may be low during night-time fasting. Relaxed wakefulness at other times of day when growth hormone and nutrient levels are high may be important for tissue repair. Laborit (1972) proposed that non-REM sleep represents increased anabolism in neuroglia, whereas REM sleep reflects heightened neural metabolic activity. The current state of knowledge seems to support the view that both night-time sleep and day-time rest periods are necessary for optimal recovery from physical illness.

Secondly, what is the effect of sleep deprivation? Williams *et al.* (1967) selectively deprived healthy subjects of different stages of sleep using stimuli that did not awaken the subject. REM-deprived subjects became anxious, insecure and withdrawn, and showed some signs of confusion. Stage 4 deprived subjects felt physically uncomfortable, withdrawn and concerned over vague physical complaints and changes in bodily feelings. Could sleep deprivation play a part in the continued discomfort and apathetic feeling of 'cured' patients?

Some stages of sleep are potentially dangerous for some patients. Hemenway (1980) reviews research on the incidence of cardiac arrhythmias and angina during different stages of sleep and their purported association with parasympathetic domination during non-REM sleep and sympathetic domination during REM sleep. In fact, the rate and degree of change of cardiorespiratory function during REM sleep and the lowering of the rate of metabolism during non-REM sleep are both potentially life-threatening. Monitoring and disturbance of patients at risk increase the chance of survival at the cost of sleep disturbance and deprivation. The so-called 'intensive care syndrome' shows a remarkable similarity between the experimentally sleep-deprived patient and the sleep-disturbed seriously ill patient, (Helton *et al.*, 1980). The extent to which pathology, liable in itself to alter mental status, is controlled for in these studies probably accounts for differences in the percentage of patients found to develop intensive care syndrome. However, team planning of care and reduction of extraneous noise can ensure longer spans of undisturbed sleep and one or two nights' recovery sleep are usually sufficient to dispel the gross symptoms. It is important, therefore, that when such patients are no longer at mortal risk they should have the opportunity and confidence to sleep undisturbed.

Many studies of the effect on sleep of general surgery, cardiac surgery, arrhythmias and fever have been undertaken in the past two decades (Kavey and Altshiler, 1979; Johns *et al.*, 1974; Orr and Stahl, 1977; Murao *et al.*, 1972; Rosenblatt *et al.*, 1969). A problem for this type of research is that the monitoring may itself disturb sleep. Disturbance and reduction of various phases of sleep were observed both pre- and, more markedly, post-operatively with a loss of normal rhythmicity.

Following the relatively minor surgery of herniorrhaphy, Kavey and Altshiler (1979) found that patients were awake or drowsing for over 40% of the first one or two nights. Both physiological monitoring (electroencephalography, electrooculography, respiratory rate and electrocardiography) and subjective ratings of sleep were made. Consistent correlations were not found between the patient's rating of the quality of his sleep (from very poor to excellent), and either the total sleep time or the stages of sleep monitored. It required detailed questioning about recall of awakenings and light sleep to improve the covariance of objective and subjective findings. It is important from the patient's point of view that he feels he has had a good night's sleep. If, however, particular stages of sleep have been lost they need to be made up during subsequent sleep. The overall picture of the post-operative sleep was of 'restlessness', light sleep and almost complete absence of REM and non-REM deep sleep.

Kavey and Altshiler (1979) cited pain and nursing interruptions as the major causes of awakening and light sleep. They found little difference in the stages of sleep obtained between those who had had spinal anaesthesia and those who had had general anaesthesia, or between those who did or did not receive pethidine during the night, and suggest that surgical trauma itself may result in sleep deprivation and disturbance of rhythm. However, pain, including post-operative pain, is notoriously poorly controlled, and, along with a reduction in nurses' provoked disturbance, better pain control provides ample room for improving the opportunity for patients to sleep. It is the best compromise which is sought between ensuring the patient's safety and promoting sleep.

Many patients report that they sleep less well in hospital than at home. The effects of minor discomfort, hunger, noise and thirst, anxiety and communal sleeping on sleep merit further study. Day-time sleep may offset the deleterious effects of night-time disturbance. As Minors and Waterhouse (1981) remark, 'provided that he has sufficient motivation man can considerably modify his hours of sleep and wakefulness.'

Whether the motivation is provided by recreation, religion, work, travel, or the care of young babies or the sick, most humans disrupt their sleep–wake patterns from time to time. The effect of variable schedules of sleep on well-being have been directly experienced by most health professionals (Friedman *et al.*, 1971) and should give us some insight into the problems faced by the sick.

Biological Rhythms

The sleep–wake–activity pattern is a circadian rhythm; all bodily functions display such rhythmicity, with peaks and troughs occurring at intervals of seconds, minutes, hours, days, months, or years. The results of studies on healthy individuals suggest that each person has a characteristic chronobiological profile in health (Halberg *et al.*, 1972; Halberg and Ahlgren, 1979). The relationship between biorhythms and illness has been the subject of much recent research, although practical applications have so far been limited. Clinical implications have been reviewed by Halberg (1977) and Minors and Waterhouse (1981). Changes in normal patterns have been found in association with some diseases, for example hypertension (Aslanian *et al.*, 1978) and respiratory diseases (Connolly, 1979). Such findings may assist with the diagnosis and monitoring of the outcome of treatment.

The rhythm of adrenocortical secretion appears to govern the rhythm of some other functions such as blood cell counts, cell mitosis and urinary electrolyte levels. The onset and severity of at least some diseases is time-dependent. It seems probable that susceptibility to endotoxins and carcinogens is greater at certain times in an individual's day than at others. For example, the highest incidence of asthmatic attacks occurs about four hours before the midpoint of the subject's nocturnal sleep span, at the time when the experimental introduction of histamine causes the greatest cutaneous and airway resistance responses (Reinberg *et al.*, 1965; Halberg, 1977). The toxic or therapeutic effect of drugs, chemotherapy, and radiotherapy may be enhanced by exploiting the spontaneously occurring rhythms. The full implications of rhythmicity in the monitoring of illness and recovery have yet to be completely explored. Provided that fluctuations in vital signs such as heart-rate, temperature and blood pressure remain within the range of normality, underlying circadian rhythms are rarely noted. Indeed, differences in the precision with which different people and different instruments measure these signs may conceal or confound cyclic changes altogether. Alterations in these variables occasioned by pathology are generally so great that the existence of an underlying rhythm may make little or no difference to decisions about care. However, for some values, what is acceptable at one time of day might be unacceptably high or low at another (Delea, 1979).

The synchronization of various rhythms is affected not only by internal events but also by external cyclic inputs (*Zeitgebers*) such as light–dark and socially determined rest–activity cycles and eating times (Reinberg, 1966). One aspect of life for hospital patients which may have an effect on physical and behavioural rhythmicity is the imposed schedule of sleep–activity–eating. This often differs from the patient's normal pattern of living and is grossly altered by pre- and post-operative routines such as fasting and night-time disturbance. Halberg (1977) found that after three weeks on different mealtime schedules the time of day when peak levels of cortisol, growth hormone, insulin and glucagon occurred was altered. Weight gain or loss differed according to the time of day the meal was taken. Is any part of the malaise of patients during and following hospitalization attributable to dissociation of previously synchronized rhythms by the disruption of habitual patterns of eating and sleeping? Grouping of patients according to age and enabling night-shift workers, and late and early risers, to retain their normal pattern of activity when cared for communally may be both physically and psychologically important for optimal recovery rate. However, Leddy (1977) did not demonstrate a shift in blood pressure or temperature rhythms following a one-hour shift of sleep time for seven days. Findings will depend upon the extent of and the number of days over which the change in activity pattern persists. Chronobiology and its medical applications seem set to have an increasing impact on the diagnosis, treatment and care of illness over the next decade.

In summary, research suggests that return to health is not solely a matter of recovering from the specific illness, but also of recovering from the effects of changed patterns of living which accompany illness—inactivity, sleep disturbance and possibly alteration in biorhythmicity. Efforts to minimize these changes during illness and advice to resume normal patterns of living during convalescence may hasten recovery and increase the number of patients who say 'the treatment was successful and I feel well'.

References

Aniansson, A. (1978). Muscle function in old age. *Scandinavian Journal of Rehabilitation Medicine Supplement,* **6**, 43–49.

Aslanian, N. L., Astrian, D. J., and Bagdassarian, R. A. (1978). Circadian rhythms of electrolyte secretion in hypersensitive patients and healthy subjects. *Chronobiologia,* **5**, 251-262.

Asher, R. A. J. (1947). The dangers of going to bed. *British Medical Journal,* **ii**, 967.

Bartlett, F. C. (1953). Psychological criteria of fatigue. In W. F. Floyd and A. T. Welford (Editors), *Symposium on Fatigue*. Lewis, London.

Bollet, A. J., and Owen, S. (1973). Evaluation of nutritional status of selected hospitalized patients. *American Journal of Clinical Nutrition*, **26**, 931.

Bradshaw, E. G. (1981). Recent advances in pre-operative assessment and pre-medications. *Hospital Update,* Sept., Vol 23 no. 5, 873–879.

Brouha, L. (1960). *Physiology in Industry.* Pergamon Press, Oxford.

Browse, N. L. (1965). *The Physiology and Pathology of Bedrest.* C. C. Thomas, Springfield, Il.

Butler, R. N. (1979). Guest editorial. *Sleep,* **1**, 219–220.

Cameron, C. (1973). A theory of fatigue. *Ergonomics,* **16**, 633–648.

Colquhoun, W. P. (Editor) (1971). *Biological Rhythms and Human Performance.* Academic Press, London, New York.

Colquhoun, W. P. (Editor) (1972). *Aspects of Human Efficiency. Diurnal Rhythm and Loss of Sleep. English University Press.*

Connolly, C. K. (1979). Diurnal rhythms: Airway obstruction. *British Journal of Diseases of the Chest,* **73**, 357–366.

Delea, C. S. (1979). Chronobiology of blood pressure. *Nephron,* **23**, 91–97.

Friedman, R. C., Bigger, J. T., and Corfield, D. S. (1971). The intern and sleep loss. *New England Journal of Medicine,* **285**, 201–203.

Hackett, A. F., Yeung, C. K., and Hill, G. L. (1979). Eating patterns in patients recovering from major surgery—a study of voluntary food intake and energy balance. *British Journal of Surgery,* **66**, 415–418.

Halberg, F. (1977). Implications of biological rhythms for clinical practice. *Hospital Practice,* **12**, 139–149.

Halberg, F., Johnson, E. A., Nelson, N. (1972). Autorhythmometry procedures for physiological self-measurements and their analysis. *The Physiology Teacher,* **1**, 1–11.

Halberg, F., and Ahlgren, A. (1979). Chronobiology—1979. *International Journal of Chronobiology,* **6**, 145–162.

Hartmann, E. (1978). *The Sleeping Pill.* Yale University Press, New Haven.

Helton, M. C., Gordon, S. H., and Nunnery, S. L. (1980). The correlation between sleep deprivation and the intensive care unit syndrome. *Heart and Lung,* **9**, 465–468.

Hemenway, J. A. (1980). Sleep and the cardiac patient. *Heart and Lung,* **9**, 453–463.

Hettinger, T. (1961). *Physiology of Strength.* C. C. Thomas, Springfield, Il.

Hill, G. L., Blockett, R. L., Pickford, I., Berkinshaw, L., Young, G. A., Warren, J. R., Shorah, C. J., and Morgan, O. B. (1977). Malnutrition in surgical patients. An unrecognised problem. *Lancet,* **i**, 689–692.

Hilton, J. (1878). Rest and pain: The influence of mechanical and physiological rest in the treatment of accidents and surgical diseases and the diagnostic value of pain. *Lancet,* **ii**, 460.

Horne, J. A. (1980). Sleep and body restitution. *Experientia,* **36**, 11–13.

Jeanneret, P. R., and Webb, W. B. (1963). Strength of grip on arousal from full night's sleep. *Perceptual and Motor Skills,* **17**, 759–761.

Jestico, J. V. (1980). Night sedation and sleep. *Nursing,* **20**, 886–888.

Johns, M. W., Large, A. A., and Masterton, S. P. (1974). Sleep and dream delirium after open heart surgery. *British Journal of Surgery,* **61**, 377.

Jung, R. (1981). Nutrition. *Hospital Update,* **7**, 883–898.

Kavey, N. B., and Altshiler, K. Z. (1979). Sleep in herniorrhaphy patients. *American Journal of Surgery,* **138**, 683–687.

Kelly, M. M. (1966). Exercises for bedfast patients. *American Journal of Nursing,* **66**, 2209–2213.

Keys, A., Brozek, J., Henschel, A., Mickelsen, O., and Taylor, H. L. (1950). *The Biology of Human Starvation.* University of Minnesota Press, Minneapolis.

Kottke, F. J. (1966). The effects of limitation of activity upon the human body. *Journal of the American Medical Association,* **196**, 118–122.

Kyei-Mensah, K., and Thornton, J. A. (1974). The incidence of medical disease in surgical patients. *British Journal of Anaesthetics,* **46**, 570–574.

Laborit, H. (1972). *Research Communications in Chemical Pathology and Pharmacology,* **3**, 349.

Leddy, S. (1977). Sleep and phase shifting of biological rhythms. *International Journal of Nursing Studies,* **14**, 137–150.

Minors, D. S., and Waterhouse, J. M. (1981). *Circadian Rhythms and the Human.* John Wright, Bristol.

Murao, S., Harumi, K., Karayama, S., Mashima, S., Shimomura, K., Muragama, M., Marsuo, H., Yarnamoto, H., Kuto, R., and Chen, C. (1972). All night polygraphic studies of nocturnal angina pectoris. *Japanese Heart Journal,* **13**, 295.

Orr, W. C., and Stahl, M. L. (1977). Sleep disturbance after open heart surgery. *American Journal of Cardiology,* **39**, 196.

Reinberg, A. (1966). Circadian rhythms. *Journal of the American Medical Association,* **196**, 108 (Letter).

Reinberg, A., Sidi, E., and Ghata, J. (1965). Circadian reactivity rhythms of human skin to histamine and allergen and the adrenal cycle. *Journal of Allergy,* **36**, 273.

Rosenblatt, G., Zwilling, G., and Hartman, E. (1969). Electrocardiograph changes during sleep in patients with cardiac abnormalities. *Psychophysiology,* **6**, 233.

Sapega, A. A., and Nicholas, J. A. (1981). The clinical use of musculoskeletal profiling in sports medicine. *The Physician and Sports Medicine,* **9**, 80–88.

Shephard, R. J. (1969). *Endurance Fitness.* University of Toronto Press, Toronto.

Simonson, E. (1947). Physical fitness and work capacity of older men. *Geriatrics,* **2**, 110–119.

Sterling, P., and Eyer, J. (1981). Biological basis of stress related mortality. *Social Science and Medicine,* **15E**, 3–42.

Takahashi, Y., Kipris, D. M., and Daughaday, W. H. (1968). Growth hormone secretion during sleep. *Journal of Clinical Investigation,* **47**, 2079.

Weber, A., Jermini, C., and Grandjean, E. P. (1975). Relationship between objective and subjective assessment of experimentally induced fatigue. *Ergonomics,* **18**, 151–156.

Williams, R., Agnew, H., and Webb, W. (1967). Effects of prolonged stage 4 and 1-REM sleep deprivation. EEG task performance and psychologic responses. US School of Aerospace Medicine. Report

Wilson-Barnett, J. (1979). *Stress in Hospital: Patients' Psychological Reaction to Illness and Health Care.* Churchill-Livingstone, Edinburgh.

CHAPTER 2

Recovery of Fitness

One of the most dramatic changes of the past decade has been in attitudes to and expectation of recovery from diseases of the heart. This vital lump of muscle, hitherto invested with mystical connections to the soul of man, is now expected to resume much of its function following infarction, coronary artery bypass and even transplant. Instead of languishing in bed for weeks and forever more regarding themselves as invalids, many such patients are encouraged to get up and walk, and within weeks of the acute illness or operation are tested for tolerance to exercise and encouraged to participate in training regimes. Knowledge gained from the huge research effort on this dramatic and emotive heart muscle has given specialist health professionals the courage to give positive advice and encouragement to this group of patients. What of the less dramatic illness and the humble skeletal muscles?

Is the level of concern about the quality of life directly proportional to the effort and expense expended on the individual patient? Early ambulation and early discharge aim to reduce complications—side-effects of being ill—and the length of the waiting list, respectively, but how systematically is the opportunity taken to advise the sick on a positive approach to living during recovery? Is the title 'health service' still largely a misnomer?

The maintenance or recovery of a level of fitness compatible with the person's way of life such that he or she can resume work and leisure activities without feeling fatigued is an important goal of recovery. Some aspects of fitness—muscle strength, flexibility and coordination—were discussed in Chapter 1. This chapter is mainly concerned with endurance fitness or stamina—the ability to maintain rhythmic movements for such activities as walking, climbing stairs, running and cycling. Loss of endurance fitness is liable to affect any person who is inactive.

Physical fitness has interested man from time immemorial. Shephard (1969) traces the historical development of fitness as a scientific concept from the early Egyptian civilizations to the 20th century. In 1946,

Johnson wrote that 'Quantitative assessment of physical fitness is one of the most complex and controversial problems in applied physiology.' However, all would agree with the proposition that an individual can work harder, for longer and with less effort when he is fit, than when he is unfit (Bassey and Fentem, 1981). Understanding of why this is so and choice of suitable physiological and psychological parameters to measure in different circumstances has been elucidated by recent research. The prestige of excellence in sport and athletic competition and concern about the deleterious effect of reduced obligatory activity in technological societies has spurred the research effort. Medical research has attempted to clarify the relationship between physical activity and the incidence of disease (Masironi *et al.*, manuscript in preparation) and health. The role of exercise in the prevention of and recovery from cardiac disease has received most attention (World Health Organization, 1968, 1971, 1972; Larsen and Malmborg, 1971; Shephard, 1981).

Shephard (1969) defines endurance fitness as 'the ability of a man to maintain the various processes involved in metabolic exchange as close to the resting state as is mutually possible during performance of a strenuous and fully learned task for moderate time (one to sixty minutes), with a capacity to reach a higher steady rate of working than the "unfit" and to restore promptly after exercise all equilibria which are disturbed.' The physiological determinants of endurance fitness were reviewed by Shephard (1969). The basic hypothesis is that the overall determinant of endurance fitness is the ability to transfer oxygen from the atmosphere to the sites of biochemical activity in the working muscles.

The exact effect of illness on respiratory, cardiocirculatory and muscle function will obviously depend upon the nature of the illness. The effect of rest alone was examined in the now classical study of Saltin *et al.* (1968). They confined three previously sedentary (unfit) and two physically active (fit) young men to bedrest for 20 days. Some resting values changed following rest: lean body mass, total body water, intracellular fluid volume, red cell mass, and plasma volume all decreased. Lung function changed very little, although total diffusing capacity and pulmonary capillary blood volume were slightly lower. The total resting heart volume decreased from 860 to 770 ml. The greatest changes were found when the subjects exercised. Comparing the responses before and after bedrest revealed that cardiac output fell about 15% during submaximal work and 26% during maximal exercise. Stroke volume was reduced and heart-rates increased during standard submaximal exercise from 145 to 180 beats per minute. Maximum oxygen uptake fell from 3.3

to 2.4 litres. Saltin *et al.* (1968) suggest that the fall in maximum oxygen uptake was due to the reduction of stroke volume and cardiac output, and that this finding was partly because of impaired venous return and partly a result of impaired myocardial function. Following a strenuous 55-day physical training programme, not only had the deleterious effects of bedrest been reversed, but the maximum oxygen uptake of the sedentary subjects had increased by 33% compared with the value before bedrest. This improvement was attributed both to an increase in stroke volume and to a widening of the arteriovenous oxygen difference. They concluded that 'the study clearly shows that maximal oxygen uptake can be altered over a wide range in normal subjects, within relatively short periods of time, by marked alteration in activity patterns.'

Many studies have investigated the effect of exercise on people who have not been put to bed for either experiment or illness. Fentem (1978) discussed the findings and concluded that in these circumstances exercise primarily 'trains' the skeletal muscles (widening the arteriovenous oxygen difference) rather than the heart. Microbiological and biochemical analysis of active muscle tissue following training has revealed increases in muscle protein, enzymes and capillaries. Scandinavian researchers selectively trained one leg or a pair of limbs, then tested the response of the heart to exercise of the untrained limbs and of the trained limbs separately. Significant improvement in cardiovascular function only occurred when the trained muscles were being used. It seems that a major effect of exercise on physical fitness is on the efficiency with which muscles extract and utilize oxygen.

The implications of these research findings are heartening for those with chronic respiratory or cardiovascular disease. Notwithstanding the fact that cardiorespiratory disease reduces fitness, such patients can improve their tolerance to physical exertion. Increase in the efficiency with which muscles extract oxygen will reduce the load placed on the ailing cardiorespiratory systems. It should alert us to the likelihood that those who have most to lose by exacerbation of their disease also have most to lose by inactivity. From time to time a patient is incidentally found to be severely anaemic on admission to hospital and yet to have been normally active up to that time. This finding could be explained by the same rationale—efficient muscles compensating for the gradual decline in the delivery of oxygen from the blood. A corollary of these findings which is of more general application is that we become fit for our habitual activities and not for other activities. The most logical and rational exercises a patient could undertake during recovery would be those which exactly or most nearly resemble the activities of his own lifestyle. If someone needs to be able to climb stairs, then the best way to become fit to climb stairs is to climb stairs.

During recovery from illness the criterion by which the achievement of the goal of fitness is judged is generally the ex-patient's subjective assessment of exertion or fatigue. Objective criteria are based on the percentage of physical capacity (aerobic power, or maximum heart-rate) which a person expends during work, or the rate at which his activity-disturbed physiological responses return to resting values after work. Objective criteria have been sought primarily in an effort to 'fit the man to the job' (personnel selection), or 'fit the job to the man' (work organization, job design) (Grandjean, 1969).

The way in which the relationship between physical capacity and work demands can be used to aid decisions about the fitness of a man for his work is illustrated by Shephard (in the press). He discusses the aerobic demands of marine surveying on elderly men as follows (Shephard, 1978a, b):

> 'The aerobic power of the average worker declines by about 5 millilitres per kilogram per minute in each decade of life. A fit 65-year-old has an aerobic power of some 30 ml kg^{-1} min^{-1} (similar in men and women) . . . Given a body mass of 70 kg, the absolute maximum intake of oxygen is $70 \times 30 = 2100$ mg min^{-1}.'

The permissible usage of maximum oxygen intake has been set by different authors at 33–50% of maximum for an 8-hour working day (Astrand, 1967; Bonjer, 1968; Hughes and Goldman, 1970). The lower end of the range is recommended (Shephard, 1974) when work is intermittent, with high peak rates of energy expenditure and adverse conditions such as arm work, heat, crawling, and obstacles to surmount. A 33% loading would reduce the allowable usage of an average 65-year-old worker to 700 ml min^{-1} . . . If a one standard deviation margin is allowed 82% of the labour force should be able to meet the standard rate of working through to retirement without undue fatigue. 'This would bring the permissible rate of oxygen usage to 560 ml min^{-1}.'

If this rationale is applied to a 70-kg person returning to work after illness, it means that he would need an aerobic power of 24 ml kg^{-1} min^{-1} to cope with that particular work without feeling unduly tired. A similar rationale has been applied to many jobs, leading to a classification of work as light, moderate, heavy and very heavy (Durnin and Passmore, 1967); and the exercise tolerance of some groups of patients has been estimated, for example those with ischaemic heart disease (Van der

Sluys, 1977). However, survey assessments of the physical strain imposed by particular jobs can only provide a rough guide for the recovery of fitness following illness. Changes in work organization, technology and hours of work make survey findings out of date quite quickly. The findings in one country or even in one firm may not apply to other jobs with the same name. The way in which individuals organize their time at work and their idiosyncratic response to particular stresses also affect the accuracy of predicting the stress–strain relationship. Ford *et al.* (1959), studying the response of 'cardiac' and healthy men to work in a steel mill, found that abnormal electrocardiograph and blood pressure responses were characteristic of the individual rather than the particular stress. Nonetheless, information about the physical stress of work and leisure activities, plus assessment of the patient's fitness, could provide a basis for setting recovery goals.

Endurance fitness tests

Astrand and Rodahl (1970) have discussed the value of and relationship between different tests of fitness, and Shephard (1978b) the problems of standardizing tests amongst different experimenters in different environments using different apparatus. The classical test of fitness is to measure the maximum oxygen uptake of a subject who is working 'flat out' on a treadmill, bicycle ergometer, or step-test. Highest values are obtained when the largest muscle groups are involved in the test, the sedentary bicycle test yielding a slightly lower value than the tests in which the whole body is moved. Local muscle and joint discomfort often cause the subject to terminate exercise before cardiorespiratory limits are reached. This maximal test is generally confined to scientific investigation on healthy subjects. Prediction of maximum aerobic power from heart-rate and oxygen consumption at submaximal work loads is more usually applied to the sick or untrained, using nomograms (Astrand, 1960) to correct for weight, sex and age. Such tests require ethical approval, a full medical examination and electrocardiographic monitoring. Whatever the test, the relationship between muscle work and physiological parameters measured is liable to be affected by the subject's familiarity with the apparatus and environment, his skill in performing the task and his motivation. Other factors which affect performance include the time of day, the immediately preceding level of activity, the time since the last meal, and, with smokers, their last cigarette. Recommendations of the ideal environment (Shephard, 1969) are that the exercise test should be performed 'in the morning, following a good night's sleep. Strenuous muscular work should be avoided on the preceding day. A minimum of an hour's rest in a comfortable environment without food or tobacco is essential and a longer period without stimulants, fatty foods, or a large meal is desirable.' He suggests that 'in hospital where a single test is being carried out for diagnostic purposes it is possible to insist upon the ideal.'

The potential risk of overstressing a sick person and the necessity of electrocardiographic monitoring during maximal and submaximal tests of aerobic power have led to a search for other tests of fitness. Significant correlations between resting parameters such as haemoglobin, resting heart-rate and heart size, and maximum aerobic capacity unfortunately do not enable a prediction of one from the other as the standard deviation from the regression line is large. The error of prediction for an individual could therefore be high. Also, such resting parameters indicative of fitness can also indicate pathology.

In many circumstances, including assessment of recovery, the aim of physical fitness testing is to inform patients of their work tolerance and to motivate them to exercise rather than measure their absolute maximum capacity. Walking or cycling at a rate chosen by the patient, keeping within some relevant symptom limit such as 'shortness of breath', angina (Borg *et al.*, 1980), or musculoskeletal discomfort, can be useful both in estimating fitness and in encouraging effort. Measurements of the time taken, distance covered and either exercise or recovery heart-rate are the type of indicators of fitness used. Such tests reduce the potential risk of overstressing patients which can happen when work loads are imposed by the observer. Bassey *et al.* (1976) describe one such test of 'self-paced walking' suitable for elderly or frail patients. Subjects were asked to walk two laps of an indoor course of 128 metres on three occasions. They walked at a pace which corresponded with the instructions (1) rather slowly, (2) at a normal pace, neither fast nor slow, and (3) rather fast but without over-exerting yourself, and they rested for 5 minutes after each walk. Speed, electrocardiogram and footfall were recorded. To evaluate the test, subjects also performed a submaximal work test on a bicycle ergometer. The results of the two types of test were compared and the walking assessment was found to correlate moderately well (correlation coefficient $r = 0.79$, $p > 0.001$) with the standard bicycle test. The use of simple self-paced tests does not remove the need to standardize test conditions, as the environment, time of day, eating, sleeping and smoking will affect the findings.

Borg (1962) investigated the relationship between objective measurements of physical performance and performance capacity with the subjective perception of exertion, and he developed an RPE scale (Rating of Perceived Exertion). This scale has subsequently been validated (Borg, 1972; Borg and Ohlsson, 1975; Borg *et al.*, 1975) and used in many studies of exercise and fitness. It consists of number ratings from 6 to 20 with verbal descriptions of alternate numbers such that 7 is 'very, very light', 13 'somewhat hard', and 19 'very, very hard'. Gamberale (1972) compared heart-rate, oxygen uptake and blood lactate concentration with RPE and found that heart-rate and RPE were related in a fairly linear way irrespective of the kind of exercise undertaken. Stamford (1976) and Bar Or *et al.* (1972) drew similar conclusions from their studies, finding that RPE was closely related to submaximal heart-rate and workload, with a heart-rate of 108–114 beats per minute corresponding to RPE 11, 'fairly light', and 147–148 beats per minute indicating something between RPE 15 and 17, 'hard' and 'very hard'. The confirmation of a reliable relationship between exercise heart rate and subjective effort is useful in enabling individuals to assess their own fitness without resorting to pulse measurement. Accurate manual pulse counting during exercise is generally impossible, both for an assessor and the person exercising, and rates above about 120 beats per minute are extremely difficult to count.

Assessment of fitness can also be made using the subjective ratings of 'muscular strength' and 'endurance capacity'. This scale requires the person to tick a number on a 13-point scale ranging from 1, 'extremely low', to 13, 'extremely high', thus attempting to compare him- or herself with others of the same age and sex. Comparing this subjective scaling with physiological fitness measurements, Bassey *et al.* (1973) suggest that changes in objective fitness status are fairly accurately estimated subjectively.

In addition to the range of objective and subjective measurements of endurance fitness, it is sometimes relevant to measure other aspects of fitness such as muscle strength, lung volumes, and heart-rate and blood pressure response to postural change, as illness and bedrest are particularly liable to alter these parameters.

Fitness and Illness

A few studies have investigated the relationship between activity, fitness and illness. Bassey *et al.* (1973) looked at changes in fitness of patients undergoing menisectomy who followed two different post-operative activity schedules. Group 1 were confined to bed for 14 days before undergoing rehabilitation and physiotheraphy, and Group 2 were confined to bed for four days, were mobile at home for ten days in a plaster cast, and then returned to hospital for physiotherapy. Bassey *et al.* found a significant increase in exercise tachycardia at a standard oxygen consumption of 1.2 litres per minute after bedrest of both four and 14 days. The changes were reversed by 14 days of rehabilitation and physiotherapy and less markedly by ten days of ambulation at home. They suggest that the changes after 14 days' bedrest may be due to myocardial and skeletal muscle deconditioning, associated perhaps with some impairment of venous return, whereas the change after operation and four days' bedrest are more likely to be due to a decrease in plasma volume and the influence of the operative procedure.

Carswell (1975) measured the aerobic power of male patients (24–45 years) undergoing vagotomy and pyloroplasty who remained in bed for two days post-operatively and were discharged after seven days. She found a 20% drop in aerobic power on the fourth post-operative day with a return to 96% of pre-operative values after a further six days. The pre-operative values were reached at about 31 days.

Carswell *et al.* (1978) investigated the relationship between pre- and post-operative fitness of patients undergoing abdominal surgery. They compared the fitness status of two groups — one with high and the other with low aerobic power before surgery. The unfit group scored 46% higher in their coronary risk factor assessment (which comprised electrocardiogram, blood lipids, blood pressure and case history) than the fit group. Despite the fact that a greater fall in aerobic performance after surgery was found in the fit than in the unfit group, the maximum deterioration in the fit group did not fall to the highest value of the unfit group. The fit group regained their pre-operative fitness status in 30 days, whereas the unfit took 50 days to reach this state. Carswell *et al.* considered that physiological fitness as measured by aerobic power is a plausible measure of the body's capacity to cope with physical insult. They concluded that their results support the view of Claremont (1922) that 'if the patient is "run-down" and the operation is not an urgent matter, he should be sent away to recuperate before rather than after the operation.' However, if the unfit state of the patient is primarily due to a sedentary way of life, he will not improve unless he increases his physical activities.

Patients may wait months, even years for elective surgery. Do they become less fit during this time? Early ambulation and early discharge following curative surgery may obviate the most devastating of deterioration in fitness. However, patients undergoing surgery which to the health professionals is mundane and minor may be left to relatively unsupervized convalescence, and even in hospital 'up and about' and 'self-care' can result in widely differing levels of activity (Lelean, 1976).

Activity and fitness—a study of herniorrhaphy patients

An investigation was made by Fordham which attempted to find out what patients did whilst awaiting operation and how active they were during the recovery period as well as monitoring fitness status. A longitudinal study of 14 men undergoing elective herniorrhaphy was carried out, from the time of placement on the surgical waiting list until return to work. Standard tests of physical fitness were used, i.e. cardiorespiratory response to submaximal exercise on a bicycle ergometer, cardiovascular response to postural change on a tilt table, lung function—forced vital capacity and forced expiratory volume—and muscle handgrip strength. The tests were chosen to cover various aspects of fitness. They were performed at the initial out-patient visit, on the day of admission to hospital, post-operatively before discharge, and at the out-patient follow-up visit one month later. In addition, subjective self-ratings of muscular strength and endurance capacity were obtained immediately prior to objective physiological testing.

Information about habitual activity patterns were obtained in two ways. Firstly by structured interview regarding work and leisure pursuits, and by questionnaire of convalescent activities and return to work. Secondly, by 24-hour recording of electrocardiograms on miniature body-borne recorders together with self-kept diaries of activities. These 'spot checks' of activities were made on a normal working day pre-operatively, on the second post-operative day in hospital, and during convalescence.

The recall of both pre- and post-operative advice concerning activities, together with the patient's comments on the adequacy and effect of this advice, was obtained by questionnaire. Information about the patient's past medical history, smoking habits and present social circumstances was obtained by structured interview.

Collated data were statistically analysed and vignettes of individuals were used to examine the extent to which the progress of each person fitted with group findings, and to elucidate the cost to the patient in terms of time, inconvenience and disability.

Subject data

Age ranged from 28 to 68 years, fairly evenly distributed over decades:

three subjects in their 20's, three in their 30's, four in their 40's, two in their 50's and two in their 60's. Twelve of the 14 had been in-patients in the past for a variety of surgical and medical conditions, but only three had recurrent hernias. Seven were smokers when first seen in the out-patient's department; by the time of admission, two had given up and two had reduced smoking, although one non-smoker had commenced smoking 20 cigarettes per day for two months pre-operatively. Eight subjects were married and living with their wives; six were single or lived alone. No patient was responsible for the physical care of their family.

The length of time patients were on the waiting list for operative admission varied, ranging from three to 33 weeks. No patient was admitted as a medical emergency, and 13 out of 14 continued in full-time occupation until admission. The one exception was on sick leave for four months; he was an otherwise healthy young man but his occupation (baker) necessitated the carrying of heavy loads.

Occupational data

From detailed descriptions given by subjects, their jobs were classified according to predominant physical demands (Table 1). Six were employed in work that was mainly physical, five in a mixture of physical and sedentary work, and three in mainly sedentary work. Nine subjects worked over 40 hours per week, the remainder 40 hours or less. Time to travel to and from work varied from 0.5 to 4 hours, and modes of travel included bicycling, walking, car, tube and train journeys.

Table 1 Work classified according to predominant physical demands

Mainly physical ($n = 6$)	Mixed physical and sedentary ($n = 5$)	Mainly sedentary ($n = 3$)
Warehouseman	Contracts manager	Accountant
Car showroom assistant	Heavy-vehicle driver	Personnel officer
Builder	Merchant Navy officer	Diplomat
Scaffolder	Stores manager	
Baker	Records producer	
Casemaker		

Leisure activities

Ten subjects pursued some form of active leisure activity, such as gardening, sport, playing with their young childrer.. However, many of these activities were voluntarily curtailed during the pre-operative period, or were undertaken at irregular intervals. Activities which persisted were those that were regarded as an essential part of the person's way of life, i.e. cycling to work, playing with children, doing housework and gardening.

Major findings

These are summarized in Table 2.

Table 2 Physical fitness

	Pre-op. OPD	Pre-op. OA	Post-op. IH	Post-op. FU
Exercise response				
Estimated maximum aerobic power (V_{O_2}, ml kg^{-1})	33 (7.8)*	34 (6.4)	—	26 (10.6)
Heart-rate at 75 watts (beats per minute)	—	106 (14)	—	125 (20)
Self-rating				
Muscular strength	7.9 (1.5)	8.1 (1.2)	4.3 (1.7)	6.8 (1.4)
Endurance capacity	7.5 (2.1)	8.0 (1.7)	4.5 (2.3)	7.2 (2.1)

* Standard deviation in parentheses.
Pre-op. OPD = first out-patient visit.
Pre-op. OA = on admission.
Post-op. IH = in hospital the day before discharge.
Post-op. FU = out-patient follow-up visit one month after operation.

Pre-operative findings

Physical fitness as measured by cardiorespiratory response to exercise did not deteriorate during the time on the waiting list, nor did the response to postural change or muscular grip strength. These findings are consonant with the continued employment and minimal reduction in activities reported by the patients. There was a small improvement in lung function between initial out-patient visit and admission, partially attributable to reduction or cessation of cigarette smoking by four of the subjects.

Post-operatively in hospital

No comparison could be made between pre-operative and immediate post-operative response to exercise or postural change as sitting on a saddle made performance of these tests uncomfortable for most subjects.

Grip strength remained unchanged, but lung functions were significantly lower ($p < 0.05$). Whether this functionally important decline was due to the effects of anaesthesia or the undoubted fear patients had of wound pain was indistinguishable.

Self-assessment revealed that patients regarded their whole body strength and endurance capacity to have fallen substantially ($p < 0.001$) during their few days in hospital, from above average for their age and sex to below average.

At first glance this view is striking in a group of patients who were out of bed on the first post-operative day and were encouraged, and in most cases succeeded, in caring for their own personal needs. However, analysis of the time spent in active pursuits (standing, walking, etc.) revealed that this had fallen from around 8.5 hours on a working day to 3.5 hours in hospital, and time in bed or chair had risen from 15.5 to 21.5 hours. Heart-rates in hospital belied this relative inactivity, being slightly higher at all times of day and significantly higher, by 13 beats per minute, at night ($p < 0.01$). The high night heart-rates in hospital could not be satisfactorily explained in terms of reduced length of sleep. Six patients reported longer night sleeping time in hospital and three only marginally less sleep than at home. The depth or quality of sleep in hospital may have differed. The finding could also be due to change in fitness and a rise in 'resting' pulse.

Convalescent findings

Following convalescence of a month, patients who returned to the out-patient clinic for follow-up were able to repeat the exercise test, and it was found that there was a significant deterioration ($p < 0.02$) in predicted maximum aerobic power and increased heart-rate at a standard work-rate, compared with pre-operative levels. This reduction in fitness is not surprising considering the comparative inactivity reported by all patients during convalescence. The patients who kept a 24-hour activity diary during convalescent ECG monitoring averaged 28% of the time engaged in active pursuits compared with 39% of a pre-operative working day.

The post-operative fitness level was found to be significantly ($p < 0.05$) and positively correlated ($r = +0.72$) with the pre-operative level. There was some evidence that those who were most fit before operation were also most active post-operatively. For example, the most fit person undertook cycle excursions by the third post-operative week, whereas the least fit person was most loath to move in hospital—spending 98% of his time in bed—and remained relatively inactive after discharge.

Lung function had returned to pre-operative levels one month after operation, as had the response to postural change. Early ambulation had avoided postural hypotension at this time. Grip strength was not significantly different from pre-operative findings, although it was observed that patients with increased grip strength had used their arms and hands to lift their body weight when changing posture, so avoiding some of the strain of using abdominal muscles.

The patients 'felt' that they had almost regained their pre-operative strength and endurance capacity, though few had attempted to resume their habitual activities at one month.

Duration of convalescence

One interesting finding was that the duration of convalescence was not related to either pre- or post-operative physical fitness. Indeed, a negative, although non-significant ($p < 0.1$), correlation ($r = -0.6$) was found between post-operative fitness and duration. Time to return to work seems an intuitively reasonable indicator of recovery from surgery and it has been used as such in some studies. However, for this group of patients return to work was apparently related to the physical content of their job. Patients with sedentary work or jobs in which they could select their own activities were all back at work six weeks post-operatively, whereas patients whose jobs necessitated lifting, climbing or driving (even though some stated that they were put on light duties at first), did not return to work until between seven and 12 weeks after the operation. The purported relationship between activity and fitness leads to the following argument. The person who undertakes the most physically strenuous work is likely to be the most fit, but because both he and his medical advisers attribute the development and potential recurrence of a hernia to his activities, he is advised and/or afraid to resume his normal work.

This leads us to a discussion of the content and outcome of advice recalled by these patients.

Pre-operative advice and behaviour

Ten subjects were unable to recall any pre-operative advice, although seven of these, so to speak, advised themselves—six to take care or avoid heavy lifting, one to cut down on smoking. Two received advice from doctors regarding lifting; one of these patients was also requested to stop smoking by the surgeon. A third was advised by his general practitioner to stop work until his hernia had been repaired. One person recalled advice from his family and friends to avoid heavy lifting.

The two patients who recalled medical advice reported that the advice had been followed, i.e. they stopped lifting heavy weights, and reduced smoking. For one patient, a warehouseman, a heavy weight meant approximately 1 cwt., for the other, a personnel officer, it meant a full bag of personal laundry—9 lbs. The person advised to stop work was on sick leave for four months prior to surgery. Before this he used to jog and climb and continued long-distance walking during his sick leave.

One patient gave up his hobby of stockcar racing and wore a hernia belt—prescribed for a previous hernia—on his own initiative. Two stopped smoking and a third reduced from 20 to two cigarettes per day without recalling any advice from others on this matter.

Post-operative advice recalled

This was extremely variable, both in quantity and quality. Some recalled advice from many sources—doctors, nurses, friends and family—but two recalled no advice at all. Some recalled very specific advice and others only vague advice. It should be noted that advisors were not asked what they said, or intended saying, as this was thought liable to make them consciously careful when advising the subjects of this study, but it is recognized that recall may not fully reflect advice given.

The aspects of behaviour about which advice was recalled were general activity, lifting and driving, and overwhelmingly the advice was negative—don't be too active, don't lift, don't drive. Two subjects recalled advice from friends about coughing and love-making.

Advice about activities included 'take it steady for a while', 'take things easy for a few months', 'no standing', and 'take the lift to the ground floor'. Specific advice about lifting referred to the length of time lifting should be avoided, though no two patients recalled the same length of time and this varied from six weeks to six months. The advice was not specific about what was not to be lifted, other than heavy weights. Advice about driving was specified about the time before recommencing and ranged from two weeks to three months for cars.

The patients' comments on advice fell into three main areas. Firstly, content—those who recalled no advice or only one vague piece naturally enough commented that they would have liked advice. There were areas of behaviour not covered; for example, when to bath, how to deal with their dressings, and how to protect their wound from the onslaught of children and dogs accustomed to climbing over them. Secondly, mode of presentation—a patient who received a number of pieces of advice said that he would have liked them in writing as he forgot what was said. He felt he was not at 'his articulate best' just after the operation so did not ask the right questions, and had a long discussion with his wife when he arrived home about what had and had not been advised. Thirdly, appropriateness—a man who was advised not to drive remarked that he had no car, but if he had had he would have driven soon after discharge. Another felt frustrated by the prolonged inactivity advised.

Advice about activities

If further studies confirm that fitness is reduced for prolonged periods by inactivity following minor surgery and short stay in hospital, it would be to the benefit of patients to give them advice specifically encouraging activity before and after operation, including the few days in hospital when the most dramatic reduction in activity was observed. It was apparent from the behaviour of the herniorrhaphy patients that pain or the fear of pain was a major deterrent to both deep breathing and exercise.

Success in giving patients the courage to be active is unlikely unless control of pain is adequate. This requires the application of knowledge about pain perception and relief to the needs of each individual. Detailed assessment of pain, and logical prescribing and administration of analgesia, together with the use of other tension-relieving strategies, should make it possible for almost every patient to be pain-free. Dynamic exercise itself can relieve or avoid additional muscle and joint aches. The sense of achievement and progression toward the goal of recovery which activity can give may further reduce anxiety.

The need for and receptivity to advice was amply shown by the many patients who attempted to prepare themselves for operation without specific individual advice, and who were hungry for advice during convalescence. Both the content and the delivery of advice need careful consideration (Ley and co-workers, 1967, 1973). What, for instance, do health professionals and patients mean by 'heavy weights'—a small suitcase containing pyjamas and toiletries, half a car engine, an easy chair, a baby? We could teach patients how to lift when we wish them to minimize strain.

The fitness of the herniorrhaphy patients did not deteriorate whilst awaiting surgery. This may not be true of other categories of patients, particularly those who are unemployed or who are temporarily unable to continue work. Advice and encouragement to maintain an optimum level of activity could be helpful. Convalescent advice could lay more emphasis on positive ways in which patients can hasten the recovery of fitness.

There is no reason to suppose that the advice recalled by the herniorrhaphy patients differs greatly from the generality of advice given to most surgical patients, though in some centres positive encouragement is given to increase activity post-operatively. Devlin (1981) describes the type of encouragement and advice likely to be received by surgical patients. He cites the risk of thrombosis and chest infection as hazards of bedrest and advises leg exercises in bed twice a day and cooperation with nurses when they 'try to get you up a few days after operation', and 'not to sit about in a chair all day—do some walking around'. After going home the first advice is to take life easy: 'that will probably apply for the first few weeks at home—unless you've had a trivial operation. Don't be in a rush to lift heavy things (you could cause yourself pain or even burst your stitches), or do a lot of bending or stretching, or to take violent exercise—if any activity causes you pain or discomfort stop and rest awhile.' Following each type of operation Devlin gives an indication of the time before the patient should resume certain activities such as drive, make love, return to work. The assumption made is that following days, weeks or months of limited activity a person suddenly becomes able to cope with a full day's work—that wound healing and the elapse of time are all that is required for recovery from surgery, despite acceptance of mobility as important in avoiding complications in the early post-operative period.

Health professionals and patients alike tend to associate the dramatic incident—heart attack, stroke, or burst wound—with increased exercise. Yet these events do not generally occur during mild dynamic exercise. Static or isometric exercises such as lifting heavy weights induce increases in blood and intra-abdominal pressure which may be undesirable, but it is the infected wounds and those subjected to the high-pressure stress of coughing which classically burst. Lichtenstein *et al.* (1970) suggest that much of the strength in sutured wounds is present immediately after surgery and that only a small increase in wound strength results from healing over the following months. We could perhaps capitalize on this fact by permitting and encouraging greater mobility during the immediate post-operative period. Leithauser *et al.* (1966) describe a positive and 'courageous' approach to post-operative mobility which they instituted in an American hospital. They advocated helping a patient 'walk back to health' after abdominal surgery, believing that it is harmful to delay 12–24 hours before getting a patient up, especially if the patient is elderly or debilitated. Their hypothesis is that the pathological physiology initiated by surgical trauma is one of stagnation involving blood, lymph, pulmonary gases and gastrointestinal contents, and that exercise, particularly walking, improves each. All patients who had undergone cholecystectomy, gastrectomy, vagotomy, hiatal herniorrhaphy, splenectomy, colectomy, pancreatectomy and abdominoperineal resection were included, but those with ruptured appendices, uncontrolled bleeding, recent coronary occlusion, or with non-sustaining blood pressure were excepted. They devised a three-stage procedure for major surgical patients which was instituted when the patient had recovered from anaesthesia and had a sustaining blood pressure—usually 2–4 hours after surgery.

> Stage 1: The patient turns on his side and is helped to place his legs over the edge of the bed and sit up. Then he stands on the floor. He is checked for rales and urged to cough a few times until any mucous is expectorated. After a few deep breaths the patient returns to bed.
>
> Stage 2: Following a rest of a minute or two the patient again stands out of bed and this time is instructed to stoop over once or twice in an attempt to touch the floor. The stooping lessens the danger of syncope and loosens abdominal muscle tension. The patient takes a few paces, then returns to bed.
>
> Stage 3: After a further rest of one or two minutes, the patient again gets up. This time he walks several steps—preferably to the bathroom—then returns to bed. He is thereafter allowed to the toilet with or without help, and is encouraged to walk once or twice more on the day of operation.

On the first post-operative day the patient is urged to walk once every hour, gradually increasing the time and distance to a comfortable tolerance. He continues these walking exercises until he returns to work. Unfortunately, the study does not document other milestones of recovery such as discharge date, return to work, or incidence of complications, except that the average stay in hospital after appendicectomy was 2.2 days and that for a series of 300 patients vital capacity returned to pre-operative levels within 3–5 days in the well-ambulated patients. The policy of immediate ambulation seems to have been maintained for decades, however.

Advice about exercise during convalescence obviously requires careful consideration and must be tailored to the needs of each individual. Day (1962), describing his work with convalescent patients, graphically illustrated the effect of what he calls 'spells' cast by word, deed or manner—prescriptions for inactivity followed by 'part-time living', which can inhibit recovery with a disabling fear of activity.

Masironi and Denolin (manuscript in preparation) list recommendations for physical activity of the healthy of all ages, those with cardiopulmonary disease, and some metabolic disorders including obesity. Hale *et al.* (1977) investigated the effects of exercise (four weeks' training) on patients with chronic obstructive lung disease. They found that although physiological improvement was minimal, exercise tolerance and self-confidence were enhanced. Beeken (1980) discusses the importance of physical activity in improving the quality of life and the diabetic state of non-insulin-dependent diabetic patients. Winslow and Weber (1980) describe progressive exercises for hospitalized cardiac patients, and Dehn (1980) discusses the rationale and gives guidelines for activity during rehabilitation to encourage patients to continue regular activity after discharge.

The merits of different schedules of exercise have been the subject of dispute. Bouchard *et al.* (1980) investigated the effect of the frequency, intensity and duration of exercise on improving fitness. They discuss the discrepancy between different studies as arising from differences in the initial level of fitness, number of subjects and strategy of data analysis. The analysis which they favoured revealed that 'frequency and intensity were more important than duration'. Bassey and Fentem (1981), having reviewed all the relevant literature, advise that improvement in stamina (endurance fitness) requires exercise such as walking to be 'a little harder or a little faster than is customary', 'three times a week', 'for 20 minutes'. This is in addition to normal activities and would help those who have returned to work but are finding the physical demands of life tiring.

It is often important to incorporate additional activity into the daily routine—walking to the bus, cycling to work—as for many people tremendous motivation is required to continue exercise exclusively for the reward of feeling more fit. If positive advice about activities is received and acted upon by those who have been ill, the goal of recovery of pre-operative or pre-illness levels of fitness may not only be achieved more quickly but even exceeded. A positive feeling of well-being rather than fatigue could be the outcome of illness.

References

Astrand, I. (1960). Aerobic work capacity in men and women with special reference to age. *Acta Physiologica Scandinavica,* **49**, Supplement 169.

Astrand, I. (1967). Degree of strain during building work as related to individual aerobic work capacity. *Ergonomics,* **10**, 293–303.

Astrand, P. O., and Rodahl, K. (1970). *Textbook of Work Physiology.* McGraw-Hill, New York.

Bar Or, O., Skinner, J. S., Buskirk, E. R., and Borg, G. (1972). Physiological and perceptual indicators of physical stress in 41 15–60-year-old men who vary in conditioning level and in body fatness. *Medical Science in Sports,* **4**, 96–100.

Bassey, E. J., and Fentem, P. H. (1981). *Exercise: The Facts.* Oxford University Press, Oxford.

Bassey, E. J., Bennett, T., Birmingham, A. T., Fentem, P. H., Fitton, D., and Goldsmith, R. (1973). Effects of surgical operation and bedrest on cardiovascular responses to exercise in hospital patients. *Cardiovascular Research,* **7**, 588–592.

Bassey, E. J., Fentem, P. H., MacDonald, I. C., and Scriven, P. M. (1976). Self-paced walking as a method for exercise testing in elderly and young men. *Clinical Science and Molecular Medicine,* **51**, 609–612.

Beeken, R. K. (1980). Initiating exercise programs for patients with non-insulin-dependent diabetes. *Diabetes Care,* **3**, 627–628.

Bonjer, F. H. (1968). Relationship between working time, physical working capacity and allowable caloric expenditure. In W. Rohmert (Editor), *Muskelarbeit und Muskeltraining.* Genter Verlag, Stuttgart.

Borg, G. (1962). *Physical Performance and Perceived Exertion.* Gleerup, Lund.

Borg, G. (1972). The basic 'noise constant' in the psychophysical function of perceived exertion. *Report 33*, Institute of Applied Psychology, University of Stockholm.

Borg, G., and Ohlsson, M. (1975). A study of two variants of a simple run test for determining physical work capacity. *Report 61*, Institute of Applied Psychology, University of Stockholm.

Borg, G., Edgren, B., and Noble, B. (1975). Effects of physical conditioning on perceived exertion and working capacity. *Report 63*, Institute of Applied Psychology, University of Stockholm.

Borg, G., Holmgren, A., and Lindblad, I. (1980). Perception of chest pain during physical work in a group of patients with angina pectoris. *Report 80,* Institute of Applied Psychology, University of Stockholm.

Bouchard, C., Boulay, M., Thibault, M. C., Carrier, R., and Dulac, S. (1980). Training of submaximal working capacity: frequency, intensity, duration and their interaction. *Journal of Sports Medicine,* **20**, 29–40.

Carswell, S. (1975). Changes in aerobic power in patients undergoing elective surgery. *Journal of Physiology,* **251**, 42–43.

Carswell, S. H., Holman, B. D., Thompson, J., and Walker, W. F. (1978). Acceptable level of aerobic power for patients undergoing elective surgery. *Journal of Physiology,* **285**, 16P.

Claremont, H. E. (1922). Shortening of post-operative convalescence: some differences between British and Continental treatment. *Lancet,* **i**, 427–428.

Day, G. (1962). Spellbinding and spellbreaking in convalescence. *Lancet,* **i**, 211–213.

Dehn, M. M. (1980). Rehabilitation of the cardiac patient. The effects of exercise. *American Journal of Nursing*, March, **80**, 435–440.

Devlin, D. (1981). *A Patient's Guide to Operations.* Penguin, London.

Durnin, J. V. G. A., and Passmore, R. (1967). *Energy, Work and Leisure.* Heinemann, London.

Fentem, P. H. (1978). Does exercise train muscles or heart? *New Scientist,* 26 Oct., **80**, 256–259.

Ford, A. B., Hellerstein, H. K., and Turell, D. J. (1959). A physiological study in a steel mill. *Circulation,* **XX**, 537–548.

Gamberale, F. (1972). Perceived exertion, heart rate, oxygen uptake and blood lactate in different work operations. *Ergonomics,* **15**, 545–554.

Grandjean, E. (1969). *Fitting the Task to the Man: An Ergonomic Approach.* Taylor and Francis, London.

Hale, T., Spriggs, J., and Hamley, E. J. (1977). The effects of an exercise regime on patients with lung malfunction. *British Journal of Sports Medicine,* **11**, 181.

Hughes, A. L., and Goldman, R. F. (1970). Energy cost of hard work. *Journal of Applied Physiology,* **29**, 570–572.

Johnson, H. E. (1946). Applied physiology. *Annual Review of Physiology,* **8**, 535–558.

Larsen, O. A., and Malmborg, R. O. (Editors) (1971). *Coronary Heart Disease and Physical Fitness.* Munksgaard, Copenhagen.

Leithauser, D. J., Gregory, L., and Miller, S. M. (1966). Immediate ambulation after extensive surgery. *American Journal of Nursing,* **66**, 2207–2208.

Lelean, S. (1976). Ready for report nurse. The study of nursing care. *Research Project, Series 2, No. 2,* Royal College of Nursing, London.

Ley, P., and Spelman, M. (1967). *Communicating with Patients.* Staples Press, St. Albans.

Ley, P., Bradshaw, P. W., Eaves, D., and Walker, C. M. (1973). A method for increasing patients' recall of information presented by doctors. *Psychological Medicine,* **3**, 217–220.

Lichtenstein, I. L., Iterzikoff, S., Shore, J. M., Jiron, M. W., Stuart, S., and Mizuno, L. (1970). The dynamics of wound healing. *Surgery, Gynecology and Obstetrics,* **130**, 685–690.

Masironi, R., and Denolin, H. *Physical Activity in Disease Prevention and Treatment.* WHO Monograph, in preparation.

Saltin, B., Blomquist, G., Mitchell, J. H., Johnson, R. L., Wildenthal, K., and Chapman, C. C. (1968). Response to exercise after bed-rest and after training. *Circulation,* **XXXVIII**, (Supplement VII), 1–55.

Shephard, R. J. (1969). *Endurance Fitness.* University of Toronto Press, Toronto.

Shephard, R. J. (1974). *Men at work: applications of ergonomics to performance and design.* C. C. Thomas, Springfield, Il.

Shephard, R. J. (1978a). *Physical Activity and Ageing*. Croom Helm, London.

Shephard, R. J. (1978b). *Human Physiological Work Capacity.* Cambridge University Press, Cambridge.

Shephard, R. J. (1981). *Ischaemic Heart Disease and Exercise.* Croom Helm, London.

Shephard, R. J. Equal opportunity for a geriatric labour force: some observations on marine surveying. *Ergonomics,* (in the press).

Shephard, R. J., Kavanagh, T., Kennedy, J., and Qureshi, S. (1981). Prognosis in myocardial infarction — the benefits of exercise as seen in non-randomised trials. *British Journal of Sports Medicine,* **15**, 6–16.

Stamford, B. A. (1976). Validity and reliability of subjective ratings of perceived exertion during work. *Ergonomics,* **19**, 53–60.

Van der Sluys, H. (1977). Evaluation of exercise tolerance and workload of lung patients. *Acta Tuberculosea et Pneumologica Belgica,* **68**, 183–192.

Winslow, E. H., and Weber, T. M. (1980). Rehabilitation of the cardiac patient. Progressive exercise to combat the hazard of bedrest. *American Journal of Nursing,* March, Vol. 80, 440–445.

World Health Organization (1968), *A Programme for the Physical Rehabilitation of Patients with Acute Myocardial Infarction.* Freiburg, 4–6 March. Regional Office for Europe, Copenhagen.

World Health Organization, (1971, 1972). *Evaluation of Comprehensive Rehabilitative and Preventive Programmes for Patients after Acute Myocardial Infarction.* Prague, Moscow. Regional Office for Europe, Copenhagen.

World Health Organization (1978). *Habitual Physical Activity and Health.* Regional Publication, European Series No.6, Copenhagen.

CHAPTER 3

Psychological Factors Influencing Recovery

A complex of factors determines how successfully patients recover from illness and the extent to which they benefit from treatment. If one sees illness as a crisis or extremely stressful event, as in Cohen and Lazarus's (1979) review, all the patient's resources or weaknesses will mediate the extent of recovery. Risks and threats of illness are very different for individuals, according to their experience and life expectations. It is these extremely varied responses to illness and surgery which has led to research in this area, psychological (and physical) variables being examined to determine their influence on recovery. This chapter attempts to review such studies in an attempt to identify positive psychological and risk factors influencing recovery. It will also focus on events in hospital which may have previously been unrecognised deterrents to recovery.

When discussing rehabilitation, Warren (1977) noted that to some extent everyone who has been ill needs rehabilitative care and that early attention to these needs may prevent unnecessary invalidity. He considered that the neglect for many who need specialized rehabilitation is due to the multidisciplinary nature of such treatment. This also related to the many aspects of the patient's life which affect the outcome of illness, including freedom from pain, psychological adjustment and motivation, income, housing, transport, occupation, recreation and sexual activity. However, many other factors that affect a patient's recovery can be identified and are represented in Figure 3.

As with the contribution of physical factors there is yet more controversy about which psychological factors help and hinder recovery. Work with the handicapped by Rosillo and Fogel (1970) was helpful in showing that an accurate appraisal by the patient of his prognosis was of great benefit in maximizing his effort towards this. This confirms the findings of many subsequent studies, that it is the patient's view and understanding

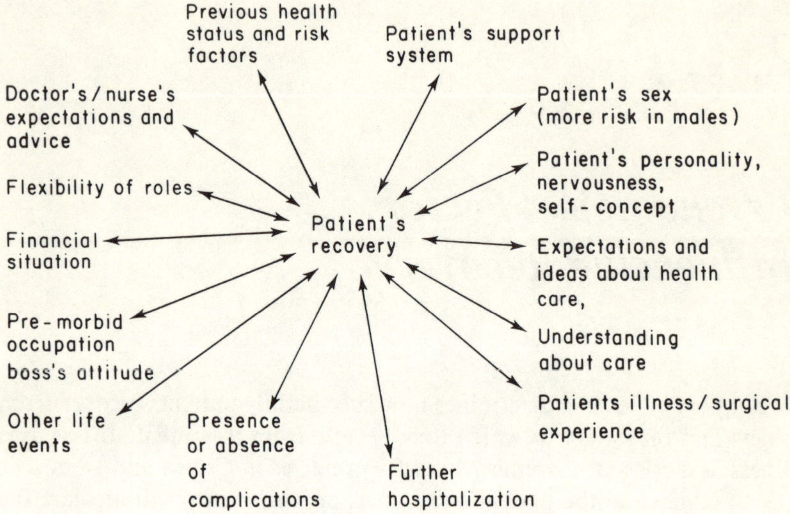

Figure 3 Factors affecting recovery

of his illness that is fundamental to his adjustment and the eventual outcome.

It is helpful to adopt Cohen and Lazarus's framework in studying patient's adjustments to major illness and how this influences recovery. If illness is the stress, the patient must adapt by:

(1) reducing the harmful environmental conditions and enhancing his prospects for recovery (by understanding what is beneficial or harmful);
(2) tolerating or adjusting to negative events and realities (to mourn the loss of an organ or good health);
(3) maintaining a positive self-image;
(4) maintaining emotional equilibrium;
(5) continuing satisfying relationships with others.

The important purpose of adaptation is to minimize and resolve negative emotional responses to illness which impede physical recovery. Coping with illness therefore involves facing a personal threat by using information and other resources to alleviate anxiety and depression. Failure to cope may lead to a complicated recovery and emotional problems. To quote Cohen and Lazarus (p. 218):

> 'There is much clinical evidence that despite similarities in medical conditions, patients differ greatly in their course of medical recovery. It is quite possible that this reflects the relative success or failure of different patterns of coping with the threats of being ill and being treated.'

The meaning or significance of an illness will obviously infer the degree of stress suffered. A major illness requiring surgery may be seen as extremely shattering to a busy mother or professional, to a lonely unoccupied widow it may not seem so terrible (see Imboden, 1972). Once the patient accepts the need for treatment and hospitalization the need to cope with future events becomes evident. The success of this coping depends on such things as intelligence, understanding the illness, charm and ability to obtain information and help from others, and in recognizing what is best to do as a patient.

Failure to cope with illness is synonymous with a reduction in all the patient's contributions and cooperation for the recovery process. The epitomy of this is the 'giving up syndrome' discussed by Engel (1962). Classically the patient is unable to accept the reality of the illness and becomes passive, unresponsive and withdrawn, waiting to die. Depression is very common after major illness and Engel sees this as a major complication to recovery.

The tendency to experience emotional distress is seen as a risk factor which may influence this response in hospital. The work of Johnson *et al.* (1970) with surgical patients and Wilson-Barnett's (1979) study in general medical wards demonstrated how trait measures of emotionality could predict those likely to experience anxiety and depression at times of stress. Cohen and Lazarus (1979) also review studies which show that a slower recovery is correlated with a higher level of preoperative anxiety and with a higher score for trait depression in nonsurgical illness.

Flexibility of coping responses to illness and treatment is shown to benefit patients' recovery. Denial during acute phases of illness after a heart attack or burns can be adaptive (Croog *et al.*, 1968). Gradual acceptance and active participation usually follows. Some patients' responses may be very changeable, according to the person present, but others are apparently persistent in their way of coping. Johnson *et al.* (1970) showed that those who believed in 'taking control' and needed information in order to do this took longer to recover from surgery. In general, it seems, patients who rely on information for their coping—'the vigilants'—fare badly when this need is not satisfied. Andrew (1967) found that extra information helped recovery in surgical patients of this type but was not so effective for others.

A positive self-image, in complete contrast to feelings of worthlessness in depressed patients, has been shown to enhance the process of recovery. Rutter's (1978) work with chronic bronchitics showed that self-perception of a strong, positive image was a persistent belief or character trait associated with more rapid recovery. Those who thought of themselves as weak and crippled, and who considered their work as 'heavy', were unlikely to manage their illness well and resume normal activities between exacerbations.

Active involvement in treatment can be seen as a particularly positive way of coping with illness. Experimental studies which encourage this have been shown to enhance the quality of recovery. For instance, coronary patients studied by Naismith *et al.* (1979) were given active encouragement in rehabilitation by a nurse and were found to reach social independence more rapidly than a control group. This was also shown in a group of burns patients by Andreason *et al.* (1972). Patients learned to adjust to enforced dependence and after a brief period of depression commenced an active approach to their recovery.

Additional stress during illness and recovery has been studied by several people. Holmes and Rahe (1967) found that a higher rate of life change was associated with an increased incidence of illness. They explained that an accumulation of stress, or need to adjust, taxed an individual's strength and he subsequently became ill. More recently, Mayou *et al.* (1978) have also shown that a poorer recovery from a heart attack is more likely when other life stresses occur during the first year after hospitalization. Nuckalls *et al.* (1972) studied pregnant women's life stress and found this in itself was not associated with a complicated recovery. However, a meaningful and close relationship, the support of a 'significant other', mediated the effect of stress. Social support was therefore shown to act as a buffer against further health problems.

Many authors, including Warren (1977), claim that general social support, financial security and occupational opportunities mitigate against delayed recovery. Lack of money, transport and comfortable surroundings may, of course, be seen as additional stresses, and their opposites as ways to facilitate a complete social recovery. It is difficult to isolate the effects of patients' previous efficient coping styles, ensuring economic stability and occupational security from the positive effects of others in providing help. Obviously an employer's understanding may be the most potent force in encouraging a rapid return to work, an event frequently used in itself as a criterion for successful recovery.

A flexible family structure with a good marital relationship is often mentioned as a positive asset for a patient's recovery. Croog *et al.* (1968), in an early review of factors affecting recovery with particular reference to myocardial infarction, discussed the benefit of a wife who could become employed as an interim measure. Mayou's (1978) team also found that a working wife could be a great financial benefit, but this sometimes caused great distress for the patient whose bread-winning status was lost.

Friendship among patients on a ward is frequently reported as particularly important to them (see Wilson-Barnett, 1979) but the atmosphere of supportive camaraderie may well be missed at home. Those with a helpful network of friends and an extended family nearby do not suffer from the emotional distress of loneliness. This could also be avoided by the beneficial effect of returning to work as Warren suggests.

Table 3 summarizes the beneficial and harmful factors in recovery. In further work with the hospitalized patient some of these factors will now be explored.

Table 3 Beneficial and harmful factors in recovery

Positive factors	Risk factors
Youth	Old age
Physical fitness	Other complicating diseases or incapacity
Good knowledge of illness	Unwillingness to know about illness
Active participation in treatment	Lack of belief in treatment
Good relationship with staff	Highly emotional predisposition
Flexible coping methods	Passive dependence
Good supportive relationships	Persistent denial
Good history of employment	Vigilant coping (when information is not available)
Financial security	Poor family relationships
Positive orientation to rehabilitation from staff	Unskilled, irregular employee
	Additional life stress
	Lack of relevant information from staff

If stress is simply defined as the need for the individual to make great adjustments to events, hospitalization can certainly be seen to demand this. The strange environment, unknown faces and threat for safety and well-being involved have been written about extensively (Robinson, 1972; Wilson-Barnett, 1979). As well as coping with illness and possibly invasive tests and surgery, patients have to master their new role and situation. Many facets of this experience are unfortunately made unnecessarily stressful by the workings of a large organization which depersonalizes staff and patients.

More specifically, patients need: information about the hospital, ward and staff; support when adjusting to threatening or sad news or events; the inclusion of family members when decisions are made or guidance is given; and preparations made for discharge with a plan for their recovery at home. Unfortunately with the everyday pressure of work in general hospital wards it has been found that these needs are sadly neglected for some patients. Evidence of this will be detailed in this section. The emphasis on patient teaching and participation has only been seen in the literature over the last decade and evidence is usually restricted to research studies rather than observed practice.

In the last two decades there have been reports that patients lack information necessary for them to understand their illness and treatment. Cartwright's (1964) interview study with patients (and their relatives) in their homes during convalescence showed that nearly half of them found it difficult to obtain information from the ward sister. Some years later the same picture emerges from other studies. Mayou's (1976) team, when interviewing 40 patients and their wives, found real concern over the correct things to do during their recovery. These people went to see their general practitioner for advice as he was 'more approachable' than hospital staff.

In medical wards, patients' needs for information were found to be most acute prior to investigations. Wilson-Barnett's (1977) study showed that diagnostic tests were the most stressful event during a patient's stay in hospital, yet few received information about what would happen. When an experimental information interview was given anxiety levels were significantly reduced. Likewise, with cardiac patients before cardiac catheterization, Finesilver (1979) found the same result when he provided two interviews at which patients were encouraged to express their fears and were given 'orientation information' about the test. These experimental patients were rated as less distressed by the nurse during the procedure and higher satisfaction with information was reported. Much of the pioneering work on designing information to help reduce patients' anxiety and cope with stressful experiences was done by Johnson. Her work in preparing patients prior to gastroscopy (Johnson *et al.*, 1973) clearly demonstrates that patients need to know how things will feel, what they will experience, how long this will last, and who will be there. Details of the actual procedure, although helpful, fail to be so effective in reducing anxiety and physical discomfort.

In general, the level of information retained by patients is not high (Ley and Spelman, 1967), and perhaps one should not assume information has not been given, or not given in a comprehensible or meaningful way, because patients say they have not received it. However, Reynolds (1978) showed a very high proportion of patients (55 of her sample of 104 patients) were dissatisfied by their lack of information. Hospital booklets and results of tests were not given and many patients were worried because they took longer than they expected to recover from their operation.

In order to take an active role, shown to be beneficial during recovery, patients need relevant information which they understand and retain. Information giving must therefore be effective. However, related to this, the evidence that patients are encouraged to be active in making their own decisions and helping their own recovery is obviously lacking. Doctors' ward rounds, sadly made farcical by 'medical' authors (Dudley, 1981), are frequently distressing to patients, who are talked about and not involved in the conversation, frightened by medical language and often exposed in front of several people. Raphael (1969) and Wilson-Barnett (1976) found younger patients were most upset by ward rounds.

Feelings of helplessness are obviously engendered by such events. In an attempt to demonstrate that involvement in care is beneficial to patients, Tryon and Leonard (1965) gave the information and choice on whether to have an enema prior to delivery of their baby. Those patients in the experimental group, given the opportunity for active choice, were more satisfied with the nurse and the procedure than others.

Patients need support and encouragement, as well as information. During troubles the opportunity to share feelings has been frequently reported as helpful by patients. 'Support' refers to an understanding listener, and the presence of counsellors in many situations may demonstrate this apparent universal need. However, nurses have not been found to be particularly occupied with this part of their role. For instance, in a very stressful situation where women needed both support and reassuring information, when attending a diagnostic breast clinic, nurses and doctors were observed to be inattentive to non-verbal cues of distress (Maguire *et al.*, 1980). Maguire's (1978) studies with mastectomy patients have shown how vulnerable these patients are to acute grief and later psychiatric morbidity after operation. He has also shown that nurse training has not provided the skill and motivation for trained staff to give appropriate comfort. This conclusion was also reached some time ago by Menzies (1961), and there is little evidence to suggest much change recently. In her interview study with student nurses in a London hospital, she explained how junior students were very keen to listen to and comfort distressed patients. However, this was not encouraged by senior staff, and students were not given any guidance on what to say to patients, or how to sympathize with them without becoming very upset themselves. Gradually through their first year of training they withdrew from sustained conversation with patients, adopting a task-orientation approach to their work. This is a particularly depressing insight into the pattern of care on some wards, as many patients confide in more junior nurses or untrained staff.

Far from encouraging the presence of relatives in the hospital to help patients cope with stressful episodes, hospitals have designated visiting hours and may actually exclude the spouse at times when the doctor is talking with the patient. With children, despite government recommendations, staff are apparently reluctant to involve mothers in the nursing care. Stacey (1970) also found that a mother's or patient's anxiety on admission could be avoided by a previous interview giving information about the admission procedure and the ward. Further work to assess the effect of 'sharing stress' with a loved one needs to be done.

Part of the information which patients and their relatives need to help them with recovery involves advice about activities at home, the likely consequences or minor problems that might occur after surgery, and an understanding of their disorder and further treatment. As Mayou *et al.* (1976) found, there is a real need for an interview with both the patient and their spouse, to allay fears, clarify misunderstandings and give an optimistic appraisal of the likely recovery for that patient. Overprotection from the spouse is very likely, particularly after a heart attack, and this may be avoided through careful discussion.

One of the major deterrents to patients coping with their recovery at home is the lack of planning prior to their discharge from hospital. The rush to empty beds for further admissions and the generally low priority given to patients' discharge arrangements are cause for concern to those interested in rehabilitation. The Royal Commission survey (1979) found 12% of their patient sample had insufficient time to make arrangements to get home. More serious neglect for discharge planning was shown by Roberts (1975), ward sisters placing this at the bottom of their list of priorities. This is then reflected in patients' ignorance about their drugs, and subsequent non-compliance. This is unproductive since, as Ferguson (1961) discovered, 10% of all admissions were due to patients' failure to cope at home through lack of understanding and adherence to medications.

Patients unfulfilled needs after discharge from hospital were examined by Hockey (1968). She found that definite nursing procedures, such as injections or dressings, were actually arranged. It was the patients' needs for reassurance, minor nursing care items and for domestic assistance that were not met. She considered that more anticipation of such needs by ward staff could avoid many of their patients' worries at home.

For the post-operative patient, whose stay in hospital is getting shorter, more of the recovery period occurs at home. It is not enough to give them a few dressing packs and an out-patient appointment for four weeks. They need to know how they will feel, especially how tired they will feel, when their scar will be completely strong, when it will cease to be hard and lumpy, what they should eat, how much they should do, and many more details. Their family, too, should be given realistic guidance on what is reasonable to expect for the duration of recovery and how to help this process (see Wilson-Barnett and Turton, 1981).

One of the essential messages to convey to patients is the individuality of every person's recovery. Every patient has a right to recover in his or her own time! Youth, enthusiasm and the rewards of returning to school or work may accelerate recovery, while at the other end of the spectrum a slow, careful recovery may be necessary for someone who has been ill for some time. The expected and normal range of recovery time for 'straightforward' surgery is frequently surprisingly wide. Doctors and nurses often find it difficult to say what the 'average time' is. To a large extent this is due to lack of knowledge. Surgeons may be able to make a prediction from their experience of years with out-patients, but for many operations there is often only one appointment made, which does not correspond with the time of full recovery. Nurses also fail to use their experience in out-patient departments to interview patients about their recovery in order to gain more systematic information on this (see Wilson-Barnett, 1981).

In conclusion, research shows that several factors affect recovery and that many negative influences are brought to bear by hospital treatment. Stress in hospital is often unnecessary and may provide a poor start to recovery. From the studies presented in this book more information should be available for improving care.

Theorists in nursing such as Orem (1971) have seen the nurse as the person responsible for helping the patient cope with illness and recovery, who gives them the support and resources necessary. It seems that the profession must face a considerable challenge in education and motivation to function more effectively. Ninety-five per cent of nurses work in hospitals, which may account for their lack of understanding for patients' needs at home. However, hospital care must be seen as only one stage in treatment, the more essential goal being the preparation of patients for their recovery at home.

References

Andreason, N. J. C., Noyes, R., and Hartford, C. E. (1972). Influencing adjustments of burns patients during hospitalization. *Psychosomatic Medicine,* **34**, 517–525.

Andrew, J. M. (1967). Coping styles, stress-relevant learning and recovery from surgery. *Ph.D. Dissertation.* University of California, Los Angeles.

Cartwright, A. (1964). *Human Relations and Hospital Care.* Institute of Community Studies, Routledge and Kegan Paul, London.

Cohen, F., and Lazarus, R. S. (1979). Coping with the stresses of illness. In G. C. Stone, F. Cohen and N. E. Adler (Editors), *Health Psychology—A Handbook.* Jossey-Bass, Washington.

Croog, S. H., Levine, S., and Lurie, Z. (1968). The heart patient and the recovery process. A review of the directions of research on social and psychological factors. *Social Science and Medicine,* **2**, 111–164.

Dudley, H. (1981). The myth of the bedside round. *World Medicine,* **17**, 53–54.

Engel, G. L. (1962). *Psychological Development in Health and Disease.* Saunders, Philadelphia.

Ferguson, T. (1961). After care of the hospitalised patient. *British Medical Journal,* **i**, 1242–1244.

Finesilver, C. (1979). Preparation of adult patients for cardiocatheterisation and coronary cineangeography. *International Journal of Nursing Studies,* **16**, 211–221.

Hockey, L. (1968). *Care in the Balance.* Queen's Institute of District Nursing, London.

Holmes, T. H., and Rahe, R. H. (1967). The social readjustment rating scale. *Journal of Psychosomatic Research,* **11**, 213–218.

Imboden, J. B. (1972). Psychosocial determinants of recovery. *Advances in Psychosomatic Medicine,* **8**, 142–155.

Johnson, J. E., Dabbs, J. M., and Leventhal, H. (1970). Psychosocial factors in the welfare of surgical patients. *Nursing Research,* **19**, 18–29.

Johnson, J. E., Morrissey, J. F., and Leventhal, H. (1973). Psychological preparation for an endoscopic examination. *Gastrointestinal Endoscopy,* **19**, 180–182.

Ley, P., and Spelman, M. (1967). *Communicating with the Patient.* Staples Press, St. Albans.

Maguire, G. P. (1978). The psychological effects of cancers and their treatments. In R. Tiffany (Editor), *Oncology for Nurses,* Vol.2. Allen and Unwin, London.

Maguire, G. P., Tait, A., and Brooke, M. (1980). A conspiracy of pretence. *Nursing Mirror,* **150**, 17–19.

Mayou, R., Williamson, B., and Foster, A. (1976). Attitudes and advice after myocardial infarction. *British Medical Journal,* i, 1577–1579.

Mayou, R., Foster, A., and Williamson, B. (1978). Psychosocial adjustment in patients one year after myocardial infarction. *Journal of Psychosomatic Research,* 22, 447–453.

Menzies, I. E. P. (1961). *The Functioning of Social Systems as a Defence against Anxiety.* Tavistock Publications, London.

Naismith, L. D., Robinson, J. F., Shaw, G. B., and Macintyre, M. M. (1979). Psychological rehabilitation after myocardial infarction. *British Medical Journal,* **i**, 439–441.

Nuckalls, L. B., Cassel, J., and Kaplan, B. H. (1972). Psychosocial assets, life crises and the prognosis of prognosis. *American Journal of Epidemiology,* **95**, 431–444.

Orem, D. E. (1971). *Nursing: Concepts of Practice.* McGraw-Hill, New York.

Raphael, W. (1969). *Patients and their Hospitals.* King Edward Fund for London.

Reynolds, M. (1978). No news is bad news: patients' views about communication in hospital. *British Medical Journal,* **i**, 1673–1676.

Roberts, I. (1975). *Discharged from Hospital.* Royal College of Nursing, London.

Robinson, L. (1972). *Psychological Aspects of the Care of Hospitalized Patients.* F. A. Davis Co., Philadelphia.

Rosillo, R. H., and Fogel, M. L. (1970). Correlation of psychologic variables and progress in physical rehabilitation: 1. Degree of disability and denial of illness. *Archives of Physical Medicine and Rehabilitation,* **51**, 227–232.

Royal Commission on the National Health Service (1979). *Patients' Attitudes to the Hospital Service.* Research Paper No.5. H.M.S.O., London.

Rutter, B. M. (1978). Psychological aspects of chronic bronchitis. *Ph.D. Thesis.* University of London.

Stacey, M. (1970). *Hospitals, Children and Their Families.* Routledge and Kegan Paul, London.

Tryon, P. A., and Leonard, R. C. (1965). Giving the patient an active role. In J. K. Skipper and R. C. Leonard (Editors), *Social Interaction and Patient Care.* Lippincott, Philadelphia, pp. 120–127.

Warren, M. D. (1977). The need for rehabilitation. In S. Mattingley (Editor), *Rehabilitation Today.* Update Books, London.

Wilson-Barnett, J. (1976). Patients' emotional reaction to hospitalization: an exploratory study. *Journal of Advanced Nursing,* **1**, 351–355.

Wilson-Barnett, J. (1977). Patients' emotional reactions to hospitalization. *Ph.D. Thesis.* University of London.

Wilson-Barnett, J. (1979). *Stress in Hospital. Patients' Psychological Reactions to Illness and Health Care.* Churchill-Livingstone, Edinburgh.

Wilson-Barnett, J. (1981). Out-patient departments: Patients first. *Nursing Mirror,* **153**, 21–22.

Wilson-Barnett, J., and Turton, P. (1981). Two aspects of nursing care (hospital and community). In P. Simpson and R. Levitt (Editors), *Going Home.* Churchill-Livingstone, Edinburgh.

World Health Organization (1980). *International Classification of Impairment, Disabilities and Handicap.* Geneva.

CHAPTER 4

Recovery from Surgery affecting Body Image

When surgery alters a patient's appearance this may affect his or her own self-image and sense of worth and attractiveness. It is therefore likely that recovery may be prolonged and distressing. Because mutilating surgery is most frequently necessary for malignant conditions, there is an added burden of fear of recurrence for the patient and his family. Most research that studies patients' responses post-operatively documents high levels of psychological and physical morbidity, although in all follow-up studies it is constantly surprising to find that the majority of patients do eventually adjust to life after surgery and the knowledge that their future is uncertain.

This chapter will be divided into three parts, each relating to a specific area of surgery. The first two parts deal with surgery commonly performed for malignant conditions—mastectomy and gut resection with formation of a stoma. These operations obviously alter the body in an 'unpleasant' way. Recovery involves adjustment to this change, frequently occurring after emotional reactions of anxiety and depression. The third section covers a review of research on patients' reactions to hysterectomy for non-malignant and malignant conditions. This is clearly linked with the concept of femininity, and the 'uterus', like 'breast', symbolizes this aspect of a woman's self-image. The operation less evidently mutilates the body but some researchers have drawn parallels between the recovery processes. These three parts do not include reference to more recently designed surgery involving radical excision of the head and neck. Research in this area is usually limited to considerations of surgical strategy and mortality. There is one paper which considers the psychological aspects of maxillofacial surgery (Rosillo *et al.*, 1973), and proposes after-treatment 'as for other patients with chronic illness'. They do discuss areas of adjustment specific to these patients, relating to the disease and feelings of loss, to the treatment, of mutilation and lastly to being in hospital and lacking freedom and companionship. Very little practical guidance for coping with these stresses is given to staff or patients except to say that those who invest a great value in their appearance will suffer more, and those who employ abnormal defences are likely to have long-standing morbidity. Unfortunately this article typifies much of the literature on caring for the patients. The challenge here is to identify risk factors, anticipate psychological distress and to review methods to improve recovery in these groups of vulnerable patients. It is becoming increasingly evident that psychological reactions to cancer and its treatment affect longer-term recovery. Stoll's (1979) review of studies indicates that patients who 'give up' or fall into a 'hopeless' depression have more extensive malignant growth and poorer prognoses than others who actively fight the disease and have a strong will to live. The relationship between reduced immunity and such psychological problems obviously has implications for all patients, but it is of particular relevance to patients recovering from early treatment of primary tumours.

THE MASTECTOMY PATIENT

By far the most common treatment for breast cancer is excision—mastectomy. Alternative approaches of less-extensive surgery and use of either chemotherapy or radiotherapy, or both, are more rare. Research has shown that these patients are vulnerable to emotional distress at the time of diagnosis, prior to surgery and post-operatively. Work has also recently given indications for improvements in psychological care, which is needed so much by these patients. (Feeley *et al.*, 1982.)

At the initial stages of lump detection and medical consultation, a sense of disbelief and shock is experienced by patients (Maguire *et al.*, 1980a; Quint, 1963; Jenkins, 1980). This is due to the realization that the lump may be malignant and the patient's life span may be greatly reduced. Maguire (1976) discusses the responses of patients at this stage and notes that most women initially worry about cancer and possible fatality rather than the loss of the breast. The physical change after mastectomy is, however, very real and causes responses which range from horror, to shame and anger. Quint's (1963) study with only 21 patients demonstrated how these responses altered over time, reflected in interview data throughout the first post-operative year. Initial anxiety and disgust at the ugly scar subsided into depression and social withdrawal after hospital discharge. This depression was sometimes short-lived and many patients were said to be greatly helped by visits from previous patients working with the 'Reach for Recovery' scheme. Practical advice often made life more comfortable. Knowledge of a 'sleeping bra' helped to provide a good night's sleep, arm exercises helped reduce swelling, and a good choice of prosthesis gave patients confidence to go out socially.

This picture of gradual adjustment is reflected in most studies for the majority of patients. However, up to a third of patients have an unduly prolonged recovery and factors which influence this must be explored. One factor which Maguire *et al.* (1980a, b, c) have documented extensively is the inadequate support which patients receive in the breast clinic and the ward. Although this refers to British hospitals where the word cancer is never seen on a notice board and rarely used in consultation or conversations with patients, it may not be too different in other centres elsewhere. Nurses were unlikely to talk with patients, recognize distress, or help support them even when they were weeping. Doctors rarely (25% of the sample) mentioned distress, tending to give blanket reassurances, rather than asking about patients' particular worries. 'Few patients or relatives who develop psychological problems appear to get the help they need' (Maguire *et al.*, 1980c), and this is also demonstrated from detailed records of communication with patients on the surgical wards. Only one in 20 interactions concerned the patient's emotional well-being. Nurses were engaged in physical-care tasks and as the necessity for these decreased during the patient's time in hospital so did any possible interaction. Nurses themselves admitted their reluctance to talk about patients' fears and worries as they might 'open the floodgates'. They accepted that they actually avoided talking to cancer patients.

The levels of psychiatric morbidity reported after surgery for breast cancer depends on the method of assessment. In studies reviewed it ranges from 40 to 12%, but confirmation that this is probably higher than for other surgery was reported by Ray (1977). She compared the post-operative recovery of 30 pairs of patients, half after mastectomy and the remainder after cholecystectomy. Patients were interviewed not less than 18 months post-operatively, to assess long-term recovery. Mastectomy patients were therefore interviewed 18 months to five years after surgery; despite this, their anxiety and depression scores were higher than the cholecystectomy patients. Although the self-esteem and extroversion scores of mastectomy patients tended to be lower, measures of social warmth, social abrasiveness and attractiveness revealed no differences. Over half the mastectomy patients still expressed concern about the loss of their breast, saying they no longer felt normal and described the operation as 'obscene'. It was these women who were also shown to be significantly more depressed.

Follow-up studies may also reveal different patterns of recovery due to the wide range of post-operative time for patients' interviews (as in Ray's study), and it seems that the longer the follow-up is the lower the level of psychiatric illness. A systematic one-year follow-up of 75 mastectomy patients and 50 control patients who had non-malignant lumps revealed much higher levels of pathological anxiety and depression in mastectomy patients (Maguire *et al.*, 1978). Psychiatric assessments of key symptoms were rated on four-point scales during follow-up interviews at four months and one year. Over half the mastectomy patients expressed some degree of anxiety and depression at four months in contrast to a third in the control group. These proportions changed little over the year, 27% of mastectomy patients persistently experiencing moderate or severe anxiety and 19% similar levels of depression. A third of mastectomy patients had severe or moderate sexual problems. Overall, 39% of this group had mood disturbance and sexual problems severe enough to warrant psychiatric help and this applied to only 12% of the controls. However, only eight patients had actually consulted their GPs in this regard.

There are studies which refute this level of gross psychological disturbance after mastectomy. For instance, Morris *et al.* (1977) studied women at two years after surgery and found no difference in social adjustment between a mastectomy group and those with a benign tumour, although 30% of all patients had 'distress'. It was stated that problems in recovery could, in a quarter of the patients, be identified pre-operatively. In Jenkins' (1980) study, 23 pairs of mastectomy patients and age-matched controls were compared on self-concept and body-image measures, and no differences were found. Patients had had surgery between three and 48 months previously and were found to be well-adjusted, only one patient reporting feelings of depression. However, this was based on non-systematic assessment at interview after other psychological measuring instruments had been completed.

It is important to attempt an identification of risk factors influencing psychological problems. Most authors are in agreement that previous treatment for psychiatric illness, youth, a high investment in one's own body and femininity, little close support, physical complications, and treatment with radiation and cytotoxic therapy predispose to a poorer recovery. The distinguishing feature with this surgery is, of course, the sexual connotations of the breast. Derogatis (1980) discusses the importance of self-image and how central the breast is to one's sexual identity. The woman with a role determined by her ability to function as a wife and mother may be more threatened by the loss of a breast. In contrast, the current emancipation to more male occupations or less sex-linked work (the androgenous gender role) may mitigate against such a threat. The impression that one's body makes to others—the reflected perceptions of others—is central to how one forms a self-image. If this is confidently established in youth, it is considered as a healthy component and a positive asset in adjustment to illness and surgery. Derogatis recognizes that mastectomy threatens the female roles of many who are likely to make a poor recovery. Related to this, a balanced pre-morbid personality and a low neuroticism trait (Morris *et al.*, 1977) are also beneficial to recovery. Close family, sex and work relations are also seen positively by most authors. The spouse's reaction may, of course, cause added concern for the patient if he recognizes that he is also unable to cope with her disfigurement. Maguire (1976) discusses how many patients would not show their scar to their husbands, would sleep separately and how one third had not resumed a satisfactory sexual relationship. The husband's attitude was frequently commented on by patients in studies. Women were frightened by how their husbands would react, whether they would lose interest in them, yet they could not initiate the necessary interaction and affection which was so needed to restore their own confidence. Husbands were generally not involved in research and seemed to be excluded from the staff's attention. They were therefore lacking the necessary guidance and support to facilitate a restoration of their marital relationship and encouragement to show affection and to reassure their wives.

Physical problems also compounded recovery. Pain was frequently reported in the muscle wall (Quint, 1963; Maguire, 1976) and this made women fearful of a recurrence of malignancy. Arm swelling and stiffness was also mentioned. However, one of the most often quoted patient responses to surgery was the appearance of the scar—so 'jagged', 'blue' and 'long'. The ugliness seemed to be shocking to patients and to be a major reason for concealment subsequently.

Clothing and choice of prosthesis are also discussed in most articles by nurses and mastectomy associations. Patients seem to need a great deal of assistance in this area. Reports of inadequate guidance are still in evidence (Seefeld, 1980; *Lancet*, 1972; Feeley *et al.*, 1982).

Perhaps one of the greatest problems for recovery from mastectomy arises from patients' inability to express problems and seek help. This may well be due to a lack of invitations or understanding from staff and to a fear of psychiatry. It is unfortunate and should be rectified in the light of a growing body of research which supports the value of expression of emotion and early treatment for depressive mood states. Recent research (reviewed below) has also evaluated changes in treatment, both physical and psychological.

Patients' psychological reactions to cancer are thought to influence their prognosis. Depressive predisposition (or a previous history of taking medication for depression) was found by Stoll (1976) to be associated with more advanced tumours. This may mean that people who characteristically suffer from depressive responses also react to cancer in this way, which reduces their chances of survival. Greer *et al.* (1979) also found that feelings of helplessness were associated with a poorer outcome after mastectomy than for others who 'fought back' or denied the threat. In this five-year multidisciplinary study, 69 patients were interviewed pre-operatively, three months after surgery and then annually. The poor recoverers, the 'stoic acceptors' or 'helpless' group had significantly more growth recurrences than the 'deniers' or fighters. However, these results have not been replicated and other research is contradictory. For instance, Derogatis *et al.* (1979) found that from their sample of 35 women with metastatic breast cancer, those who had more dysphoric moods and were more symptomatic overall survived longer than others who had higher positive moods and better attitudes to their doctors. Although the disease was more advanced in this study than others, certain psychological responses cannot be encouraged as a way of impeding the disease until results are more consistent. There is exploratory work to teach patients and to test the 'fighting back' approach of Simonton and Simonton (1975).

Research evaluating interventions for aiding patients' adjustment to cancer and surgery is sadly lacking, as Miller *et al.* (1976) found in their review. Practical suggestions are not lacking. One such, made by Seefeld (1980), to allow at least two or three days between biopsy and mastectomy, seems humane and necessary. From his lengthy experience this seems to facilitate early adjustment, less shock and grieving in the initial post-operative period, and a more satisfactory longer-term recovery. The uncertainty element of going to theatre for biopsy or mastectomy seems to evoke excessive anxiety pre-operatively which previous research has associated with complications (see Chapter 3). Seefeld also mentions that radical mastectomy has yet to be demonstrably associated with better long-term survival.

McDowell (1980) reports that insertion of an internal prosthesis at the time of mastectomy is usually uncomplicated and leads to better post-operative adjustment. Of 50 patients treated in this way 90% had a completely satisfactory recovery. They were said to benefit from an early outwardly normal appearance and were relieved of the suffering caused by the unsightly scar after mastectomy. (For the 10% who had wound breakdown a repeat operation was necessary.) In this centre in Ulster, needle biopsy of lumps provides an instant diagnosis and does not necessitate a general anaesthetic. Pre-operative counselling is then undertaken by a surgeon, psychiatrist and ward sister. It is difficult to assess whether the reconstructive surgery or the careful attention to patients' psychological needs accounts for the more complete recovery of these patients. However, a recent review by Ward (1981) also gives a favourable report of surgical innovation of this type.

Counsellors from associations, volunteers, and ex-mastectomy patients are generally considered most helpful with patients after surgery. The 'Reach for Recovery' campaign in the USA and the Mastectomy Association in Britain have hand-picked representatives who visit in hospital and at home. They are particularly good at giving practical hints on bras and external prostheses. Some centres (see letter to *Lancet,* 1972) recommend a prosthesis clinic where such representatives can help women, who then also gain companionship from each other.

The most extensive evaluation of a counselling service has been done by the Oxford team Maguire, Tait, Brooke, Thomas and Sellwood (1980a). A nurse counsellor was employed to support patients before and after surgery for over a year through visits at home and in the out-patients' department. The aims of this counsellor were (Maguire *et al.*, 1980b):

(1) to provide each patient with information, advice, and practical and emotional support from the time of admission until 12 months after surgery;
(2) to help each patient obtain a satisfactory prosthesis;
(3) to help each patient regain full use of the affected arm or adapt to any residual disability;
(4) to encourage early return to housework, work, social and leisure activities;
(5) to encourage early resumption of marital and other key relationships;
(6) to help each woman adapt to the diagnosis, breast loss and other treatments;
(7) to monitor routinely the physical, social and psychological adjustment of each patient, and when problems were detected which the nurse could not resolve, to refer the patient to an appropriate agency.'

Evaluation of this counsellor's effect was planned by psychiatric assessment of the patients in the experimental group ($n=75$) and in the control group ($n=77$) immediately after surgery, at three months and again at 12 months. At three months there was no difference in the prevalence of anxiety and depression between the two groups; a third were described as having either a mild, moderately severe or severe anxiety state, or depressive illness.

Sexual problems were found in the same proportion of patients. However, significantly fewer patients in the counselled group (8%) than in the control group (30%) were still psychiatrically ill at the 12–18 months' assessment. Due to the nurse counsellor's training in detecting emotional problems, more patients in this group were referred for psychiatric help, which was effective in preventing the long-standing morbidity (detected in the control group). She recognised 89% of the patients in her group who developed psychiatric problems assessed by the research psychiatrists.

Many hospitals have now developed the role of specialist nurses such as mastectomy counsellors or stoma therapists who advise patients practically but who also offer continuous support throughout the post-operative period for at least a year.

As with a very few other patient groups, the needs for both follow-up care and advice are well documented for mastectomy patients. However, as yet, our knowledge is insufficient to give clear-cut guidelines for practice. Mastectomy patients seem particularly emotionally vulnerable during the first year after surgery, and long-standing morbidity may be reduced by continuous support and psychiatric referral where necessary. More systematic guidance on physical aids seems necessary, and restorative surgery shows signs of reducing initial shock and psychological distress. Patients vulnerable to emotional problems can now be identified and this should prepare staff to give extra attention to both the patient and their spouse. In general, partners have not been counselled systematically and this offers a future research avenue.

References

Derogatis, L. R. (1980). Breast and gynaecological cancers. Their unique impact on body image and sexual identity in women in J. M. Vaeth (Editor) *Frontiers of Radiation Therapy and Oncology*, Vol 14, Karger, Basel, pp. 1–11.

Derogatis, L. R., Abeloff, M. D., and Melisaratos, N. (1979). Psychological coping mechanisms and survival time in metastatic breast cancer. *Journal of the American Medical Association*, **242**, 1504–1508.

Feeley, T. M., Peel, A. L. G. and Devlin, H. B. (1982). Mastectomy and its Consequences. *British Medical Journal*, **284**, 1246.

Greer, S., Morris, T., and Pettingale, K. W. (1979). Psychological responses to breast cancer: Effect on outcome. *Lancet*, **ii**, 785–787.

Jenkins, H. M. (1980). Self concept and mastectomy. *Journal of Obstetrics, Gynaecologic and Neonatal Nursing,* Jan./Feb., 38–42.

Lancet (1972). Letter. ii, 181.

Maguire, P. G. (1976). The psychological and social sequelae of mastectomy. In J. G. Howells (Editor), *Modern Perspectives in the Psychiatric Aspects of Surgery.* Brunner Mazel, New York, pp. 390–421.

Maguire, P. G., Lee, E. G., Bevington, D. J., Kuchermann, C. S., Crabtree, R. J., and Cornell, C. E. (1978). Psychiatric problems in the first year after mastectomy. *British Medical Journal,* (i) 1963–1965.

Maguire, P., Tait, A., Brooke, M., Thomas, C., and Sellwood, R. (1980a). Effect of counselling on the psychiatric morbidity associated with mastectomy. *British Medical Journal,* **281**, 1454–1456.

Maguire, P., Tait, A., Brooke, M., and Sellwood, R. (1980b). Planning and caring programme. *Nursing Mirror,* **150**, 35–37.

Maguire, P., Tait, A., and Brooke, M. (1980c). A conspiracy of pretence. *Nursing Mirror,* **150**, 17–19.

McDowell, P. G. (1980). Mastectomy and insertion of prosthesis. *Nursing Times,* **76**, 1258–1261.

Miller, C. L., Denner, P. R., and Richardson, V. E. (1976). Assisting the psychological problems of cancer patients: A review of current research. *International Journal of Nursing Studies,* **13**, 161–199.

Morris, T., Greer, H. S., and White, P. (1977). Psychological and social adjustment to mastectomy: a two year follow-up study. *Cancer,* **40**, 2381–2387.

Quint, J. C. (1963). The impact of mastectomy. *The American Journal of Nursing,* **63**:11, 88–92.

Ray, C. (1977). Psychological implications of mastectomy. *British Journal of Social and Clinical Psychology,* **16**, 373–377.

Rosillo, H. R., Welty, M. J., and Graham, W. P. (1973). The patient with maxillofacial cancer. II. Psychological aspects. *Nursing Clinics of North America,* **8**, 153–158.

Seefeld, B. (1980). Breast cancer. I. New approaches to treatment. Care and counselling. *Journal of Practical Nursing,* **30**, 27–37.

Simonton, O. C., and Simonton, S. M. (1975). Belief Systems and Management of the emotional aspects of malignancy. *Journal of Transpersonal Psychology,* **8**, 29–48.

Stoll, B. (Editor) (1976). *Risk Factors in Breast Cancer.* Heinemann, London, pp. 193–206.

Stoll, B. (Editor) (1979). *Mind and Cancer Prognosis.* John Wiley, Chichester.

Ward, C. M. (1981). Reconstruction of the breast after mastectomy. *Journal of the Royal Society of Medicine,* **74**, 327–330.

RECOVERY AFTER SURGERY INVOLVING THE FORMATION OF A STOMA

Bowel resection frequently necessitates fashioning a stoma to remain either temporarily or permanently after surgery. This alters the mode of defaecation in a radical way and requires fundamental adjustment by the patient. Similarly to those patients needing mastectomy, this extensive treatment is commonly associated with a malignant disorder and the fear of death complicates adjustment to a 'new' unsightly aspect of the body. The symbolic meaning of the stoma has been discussed by Orbach and Tallent (1965). They reviewed material from previous reports, noting that depression of long standing was frequently associated with the presence of the stoma itself and this directly related to patients' altered perception of their bodies as ugly. Their own interview study with 48 patients resulted in all patients seeing the stoma as destructive to their physical appearance. Accompanying this were feelings of great weakness and fragility, of being tied to the bathroom and being directed by their bodies. In more depth, the alteration to evacuation through the front of their bodies was very difficult to accept. Symbolically a bleeding pink opening was associated with the female sex and men felt feminized. The necessity of irrigation and touching a 'dirty' area was also distressing as a breach of taboo. Misunderstandings of anatomy of the gut and possible 'back-washes' also made patients confused and nervous.

Feelings of mutilation and personal inadequacy reported by Orbach and Tallent are frequently found in other studies. However, it is important to discuss adjustment in the light of previous illness and the contrasts post-operatively. Colostomies are usually performed after surgery for cancer of the large bowel, when patients have been relative fit previously, whereas ileostomies are done as the last stage of treatment for chronic ulcerative conditions of the colon. As Cunningham (1969) found from a postal questionnaire to 1273 colostomates, 978 had been ill for only a month or so, whereas of 1973 ileostomies, 269 had been ill for a month or so, 532 had been ill for 1–12 months and 634 had been ill for more than five years. Patients in the ileostomy group are greatly relieved from constant diarrhoea and begin to absorb nourishment and become strong again. However, management of an ileostomy tends to be more problematic than a colostomy. The faeces are more fluid and malodorous, tending to flow fairly irregularly throughout the day. Surgery for bladder cancer frequently results in an ileal conduit and this should also be considered as a type of ileostomy. This drains urine, but may be malodorous and cause skin excoriation. Colostomies tend to act once a day, when a normal diet is re-established and may be irrigated to control evacuation at the patients' convenience.

Research on patients' recovery after gut surgery has concentrated on adjustment to life with a stoma rather than to the possibility of a recurring malignancy. Levels of psychiatric morbidity vary with the sample and with the orientation of the researcher. The results of interview studies tend to reveal more worries and deterioration in social and sexual relations; postal questionnaires tend to give more positive results. This may be due to the sample differences, the latter type of study characteristically drawing on a membership list from an association from which the more motivated and active patients may reply [see, for example, Burnham *et al.*, (1977), and Mitchell (1980)]. The contrast in sample size is also noticeable; interviews are usually done with 50 or less patients, whereas postal surveys frequently include hundreds of patients.

The emphasis on sexual activity post-operatively has resulted not only from anatomical interest and a review of surgical techniques which may preserve essential structures, but also since it is an indicator for psychological adjustment. Bernstein and Bernstein (1966) discussed the likelihood that removal of lymphatic tissue might destroy parasympathetic and sympathetic nerves controlling erection, and the sometimes unnecessary excision of the circular fibres required for ejaculation. Rates of impotence in patients after abdominoperineal excision of the rectum varied between 53 and 100% in follow-up clinics. The authors argued that surgeons may be able to retain certain structures, thus reducing the levels of impotence without increasing the risk of tumour recurrence. For ileostomy patients these structures can be retained, and sexual activity should not be affected by physical factors. These patients also tend to be younger and possibly more inhibited by physical appearance than those with a colostomy, which can be controlled more effectively. Conflicting results exist as to the level of persistent sexual problems for ostomists, although in a recent textbook (Kolodny *et al.*, 1979) much higher rates of sexual impairment are noted for those with an ileal conduit (80%) when compared to colostomy and rectal excision (40%), and ileostomy and removal of the rectum (15%). Dlin *et al.* (1969) reported no change in overall psychiatric referral rates, or in sexual activities, for both colostomy and ileostomy patients: 22% had increased and 21% had decreased their sexual activities since surgery. (These results were obtained from postal questionnaires completed by 409 patients over ten years ago.) Two members of this same research team, Dlin and Perlman (1971), also noted how sexually active many patients over 50 years' old were, 'Most ostomists maintain an active and interested sexual life after surgery'. They recognize that men may concentrate on their ability to perform while women are more aware of how they look.

In all these studies, time since surgery was not standardized within the sample. Aspects of recovery such as social readjustment, sex and emotional responses probably change over time, usually improving.

It is important to trace patients' responses from hospitalization to discharge time, and in the longer term to understand what is involved. Few studies involve the period preceding surgery as this may be done as an emergency. By this very fact, however, colostomy and ileal conduit patients have less time to accept the results and necessity of surgery. As Jackson (1976) observed, most patients were shocked by this crisis. Although only six hospitalized patients were involved in this study, a characteristic pattern of response emerged. Patients expressed ambivalence about wanting to live, and also guilt and regret that they had not selected an alternative treatment even though they were not pre-warned about the catastrophe to come (the colostomy). It was also evident that patients had not started to adjust or resolve the crisis of the surgery and subsequent changes in body function while in hospital. From this it would appear that patients start to cope with these new events after their return home.

From questionnaire data on 36 patients' 'course immediately after surgery', Druss *et al.* (1969) learned of strong, very unpleasant reactions to the surgery in two-thirds of the sample. Twenty-two patients manifested depression by crying and negative comments about the colostomy. Younger patients suffered more from depression. The researchers were not able to predict long-term adjustment from initial reactions in hospital, but patients did comment that the faith of their doctors and nurses carried them through in hospital.

After discharge, however, stories of disability and complications were frequent. Over a quarter of these patients required rehospitalization for problems with their colostomy. The first year was viewed by most as a period of adjustment and experimentation. During this time there was a definite deterioration in social relationships in 72% of the group, usually from fear of odour. Life change was due to travel restrictions and lengthy irrigation procedures for half these patients. Obsessiveness over bowel movements and cleanliness was noted in a small number of patients and prevented a normal lifestyle. Similar morbidity was found in a study with patients at home one year later. The famous study of Devlin *et al.* (1971) found a depressive state in 25% of 120 colostomy patients and half of the sample were considerably more socially isolated than the average person. Unsatisfactory toilet facilities affected 34% of these patients and practical difficulties were very commonly associated with appliances and disposal. Twenty-two per cent of the patients were unemployed after surgery and the majority had altered their type of work, of necessity.

Longer-term follow-up studies tend to show 'good' recovery for the majority of patients, but severe incapacity in a small proportion after the first year. Notable research includes Pryse-Phillip's (1971) study with patients who had lived with a colostomy for at least 18 months. Six of the 20 patients showed high levels of depression, many physical symptoms and numerous bag changes each day. Universal reports from this sample of early anxiety and embarrassment contrasted with two-thirds of the patients coping well in the longer term. The six generally disabled people were most affected by the fear of smell and became deluded by its intensity and preoccupied with recriminations and depressive guilt. The only personality variable found in association with this pattern of poor recovery was a high neuroticism score from the Eysenck Personality Inventory.

Adaptation at home is of course related to the family's response to the surgery and their adjustment to an altered role for one of its members. In a study of 38 colostomy patients by Dyk and Sutherland (1956), details of marital relationships following surgery were described. Although this paper is not recent, few other studies concentrate on the reactions of family or spouse. It is worth noting the degree of discord reported. Only 14 spouses—eight wives and six husbands—were said to have been encouraging and supportive. Only a third of these patients had help with the colostomy from their spouse and other family members had not seen it. Seven wives had severe reactions to seeing the colostomy, which involved vomiting, fainting, or extreme fright. Husbands were not so repulsed by the sight. Wives did not receive so much help as husbands with the stoma and felt so weak that they needed help with housework 'more than anything'. Single patients generally felt they would never show the colostomy to anyone. Poor marital relations before surgery continued after surgery but seemed to be associated with great loss of esteem for the patient. Emotional support for those patients in need was certainly lacking where marital strife existed.

Longer-term follow-up by postal questionnaire to 376 ileostomy patients, gave a picture of successful adjustment for almost 90% of them (Burnham *et al.*, 1977). Levels of sexual functioning were unchanged for this sample of both men and women, although 50% of the males were impotent after rectal excision. Of these ileostomists, 12% ascribed marital tension, unhappiness or even separation to the stoma. However, the authors felt this study agreed with results of Daly and Brooke (1967), which demonstrated a good quality of life in terms of work and recreation for most of the sample.

From many of these studies it appears that psychological distress is caused by physical problems with the stoma. In one of the rare studies of patients with an ileal conduit, Jones *et al.* (1980) found major problems with leakage and skin excoriation for many patients. Social life was restricted for two-thirds (21) of the sample for fear of damaging the stoma, or leakage, or awareness of the appliance. All the males were impotent and only a third of the sample retained some sexual activity.

Problems most commonly recurring have been recorded by Lennenberg (1971) and Rowbottom (1971). Re-operation was said to be necessary for over half the patients in records reviewed by Lennenberg. For minor problems visits with further help were usually made in the first year, although a fifth of the patients returned to the clinic during the second year. Earlier visits, for both colostomy and ileostomy patients, involved poor management of stoma, appliances and techniques, skin problems, odour and gas, emotional support, social adjustment, eating problems and lack of resources. Later visits were required for new equipment or techniques, eating or skin problems, additional information and reassurance. Crises which could occur at any time included prolapse, hernia, skin breakdown, fistula or haemorrhage, severe depression and sudden inability to contain discharge. These potential and real problems obviously give due cause for patients to feel insecure and handicapped.

Rowbottom (1971) found that problems were more plentiful for transverse than sigmoid colostomies. Two-thirds of the visits were necessary for odour problems, a half for skin irritation and a third for leaking appliances. Flatus was also complained of—the noise being so embarrassing—but this is unfortunately incurable. Diet was said to be tried and tested to suit individuals.

The recovery and adjustment period is made more problematic by the need for additional radiotherapy or cytotoxic therapy. Breckman (1980) discusses this in detail with special guidelines for detecting depression of bone marrow function, which may cause the stoma to bleed, and cystitis and diarrhoea caused by cytotoxic agents which are irritant to membranes. Patients may well feel distraught about a recurrence and despair that this is necessary after their radical surgery from which they had apparently recovered.

Most researchers recognize a number of complicating factors after bowel surgery. A permanent stoma can be a means of relieving symptoms in chronic colitis, when recovery is usually shown to be satisfactory. However, the crisis of sudden severe illness and major surgery without warning frequently delays adjustment to a colostomy. Agents of support and help are said to be needed by these patients and, as with other patient groups, many are unfortunately neglected by staff and their families. Specialist nurses and firm's representatives are not universal and it is ward and clinic nurses who usually need to support and teach most patients.

From the retrospective studies on patients' views, Breckman (1980) notes the absence of sex counselling after surgery and Mitchell (1980) the serious lack of information given to families on stoma care.

In her study, Mitchell (1980) found that 90% of patients did not try to wear a bag pre-operatively and 35% did not meet a healthy, recovered ostomist, despite the fact that two-thirds of those who did have this opportunity felt very pleased. In one area nearly three-quarters of the patients did not receive a home visit from a district nurse or stoma therapist.

When discussing ideals for care, research has mainly relied on patients' and professionals' opinions in the absence of controlled study. Continuity of care—the same person giving care in hospital and at home—is approved of by Mitchell's patients, but only 17% of British nurses considered that one person should be responsible for patient teaching (Bailey, 1977). Only 21% of nurses considered they should play an important part in advising on diet. It may well be due to this type of response by nurses that some nurse specialists or stoma therapists are supported so strongly by doctors and nurses [see Jones *et al.* (1980), Rowbottom (1971), Mitchell (1980), and others]. A specialist provides continuity and knowledge of the practicalities of appliances, deodorants and diet. This information to solve problems was thought by most authorities to be a major contribution in avoiding delayed adjustment.

Stoma clinics and ostomy societies may also provide practical help and social support. Those who run clinics (Rowbottom and Lenneberg) obviously support their aims, but the associations tend to have the added component of mutual help thought to be so constructive to long-term adjustment.

As in other areas, considerable morbidity exists, frequently linked to physical and practical problems of stoma management. More progress in follow-up care seems to be evident in the literature, but teaching and guidance of patient and family (Devlin and Plant, 1979) prior to discharge tends to be inadequate in meeting an immense, possibly insatiable, need. The conclusions reached in 1971 by Devlin *et al.* still reflect today's situation:

(1) A stoma is an immense price to pay for treatment (especially if it is not preceded by a lengthy illness).
(2) often severely disabled people are not identified by follow-up care, and common factors which might identify them prior to surgery have not been found
(3) the existence of psychological disturbance is rarely diagnosed.

References

Bailey, A. J. (1977). Nursing the patient with a colostomy. *Nursing Times,* **73,** 382–385.

Bernstein, W. C., and Bernstein, E. F. (1966). Sexual dysfunction following radical surgery for cancer of the rectum. Paper of American College of Surgeons, Read at the Regional Meeting of the American College of Surgeons, Cleveland Ohio. March 16th. *Published Proceedings,* 328–332.

Breckman, B. (1980). Care of the ostomist undergoing radiotherapy and anti-tumour chemotherapy. *Nursing Times,* **76,** 1568–1573.

Burnham, W. R., Lennard-Jones, J. E., and Brooke, B. (1977). Sexual problems among married ileostomists. *Gut,* **18,** 673–677.

Cunningham, M. E. (1969). *A Demographic Survey of Ostomatists.* United Ostomy Association, Los Angeles.

Daly, D. W., and Brooke, B. N. (1967). Ileostomy and excision of the large intestine for ulcerative colitis. *Lancet,* **i,** 62–64.

Devlin, H. B., Plant, J. A., and Griffin, M. (1971). Aftermath of surgery for anorectal cancer. *British Medical Journal,* **ii,** 413–418.

Devlin, H. B., and Plant, J. (1979). Sexual function—an aspect of stoma care. *British Journal of Sexual Medicine,* **6,** 33–37.

Dlin, B. M., Perlman, A., and Ringold, E. (1969). Psychosexual response to ileostomy and colostomy. *American Journal of Psychiatry,* **126,** 122–381.

Dlin, B. M., and Perlman, A. (1971). Emotional response to ileostomy and colostomy in patients over the age of 50. *Geriatrics,* June, 113–118.

Druss, R. G., O'Connor, J. F., and Stem, L. O. (1969). Psychologic response to colectomy. *Archives of General Psychiatry,* **20,** 419–427.

Dyk, R. B., and Sutherland, A. M. (1956). Adaptation of the spouse and other family members to the colostomy patient. *Cancer,* **9,** 123–138.

Jackson, B. S. (1976). Colostomates' reactions to hospitalisation and colostomy surgery. *Nursing Clinics of North America,* **11**:3, 417–425.

Jones, M. A., Breckman, B., and Hendry, W. F. (1980). Life with an ileal conduit: Results of questionnaire surveys of patients and surgeons. *British Journal of Urology,* **52,** 21–25.

Kolodny, R. C., Masters, W. H., Johnson, V. E., and Biggs, M. A. (1979). *Textbook of Human Sexuality for Nurses.* Little, Brown and Co., Boston.

Lennenberg, E. (1971). Role of enterostomal therapists and stoma rehabilitation clinics. *Cancer,* **28,** 226–229.

Mitchell, A. (1980). Patients' views on stoma care. *Nursing Mirror,* **150,** 38–41.

Orbach, C. E., and Tallent, N. (1965). Modification of perceived body and of body concepts. *Archives of General Psychiatry,* **12,** 126–135.

Pryse-Phillips, W. (1971). Follow-up study of patients with colostomies. *American Journal of Surgery,* **121-2,** 27–32.

Rowbottom, J. L. (1971). Colostomy problems—dietary and colostomy management. *Cancer,* **28,** 222–225.

BODY IMAGE AND RECOVERY FROM HYSTERECTOMY

Christine Webb

Women recovering from hysterectomy may find their own image of themselves radically changed even though there is no visible alteration of the body such as there is for patients after mastectomy or formation of a stoma. For many women, having a hysterectomy is a profound threat to their self-concept as a feminine person—an attractive sexual being for whom child-bearing has been a major and highly valued social role.

Having a positive self-concept means that an individual respects herself, considers herself worthy; she does not necessarily consider herself better than others, but she definitely does not consider herself worse. Low self-esteem, on the other hand, implies self-rejection, self-dissatisfaction, self-contempt (Rosenberg, 1965). Self-concept results from how a person thinks others view her. While a person develops a basic self-image as part of their personality, self-concept can also be modified by particular situations and the responses of significant others. The self-concept is thus consolidated or confirmed after successful resolution of a life crisis, but may be damaged if the outcome of a traumatic event is not experienced as positive. Because a person's self-concept is a social phenomenon, supportive networks of family and friends may strengthen resistance by providing validation of self-worth in the face of challenges which could tend to lower self-esteem (Garrity *et al.*, 1977).

Self-concept derives partly from the value given to the social roles people play. Those who hold highly valued roles will tend to derive their self-esteem from these and may feel devalued if they lose them. This can be the case when people lose their jobs (Gore, 1978) and, in cultures where women's reproductive functions are highly valued, a hysterectomy may lead to similar effects. The woman has lost her main role in life and feels less valued as a consequence. Those around her may convey, by their words and actions, that they too value her less.

Hysterectomy has been described as a 'surgical disruption to the self-concept of "Femininity" ' (Wolf, 1970). Because of its part in menstruation and childbirth, the uterus may be seen as central in the formation of attitudes towards body image, social role and gender role. Women may see themselves as defeminized after this operation, and how they react afterwards will be strongly influenced by the quality of support given by their sexual partners.

Femininity has been linked with reproductive wholeness in a great many cultures and historical periods. In those societies and social classes, where women are more exclusively valued as bearers of children than in others, they are more likely to suffer depression if they are childless or wombless (Notman, 1976). A shift away from the domestic and child-bearing role as a central focus of women's status and self-concept as more women take to paid work outside the home may therefore bring changes in the emotional meaning of hysterectomy.

Sexuality is central rather than subordinate in the impact of breast and gynaecological cancers in Derogatis's opinion (Derogatis, 1980). These conditions can devastate a woman by imposing a unique threat to her self-concept and psychological integration, and gender role definition is a powerful mediating influence on her adjustment. The highly 'feminine' female is often at greater risk in that her personal role posture tends to be rigid, and her expectation of her partner's behaviour is also inflexible (Derogatis, 1980).

Studies of recovery from hysterectomy report many old wives' tales which are part of popular folklore and which may become self-fulfilling prophecies for women and their partners. 'If you don't have a womb, you're not a woman' (Wolf, 1970) sums up the evaluation of women principally in terms of their reproductive functions. Some myths focus on loss of physical attractiveness and fear of masculinization as a result of the operation. One woman in Raphael's study (Raphael, 1972) fantasized that she was growing a beard, and saw herself as failing in all her feminine role functions. Some women remarked 'you are never the same again' (Raphael, 1972).

'Wholeness' is threatened for some women (Williams, 1976) and they may feel that 'everything is taken away' including femininity and sexuality. Feelings of mutilation, deprivation and resentment may occur (Thompson, 1975).

The best part of the operation for some women is 'getting rid of the curse' (Raphael, 1972). Others, however, regret the loss of menstruation because for them it has represented a 'monthly cleaning out' (Raphael, 1972).

Partners of women undergoing hysterectomy have sometimes heard what could be called 'old husbands' tales'. Wolf (1970) considers that many of these men have a great deal of anxiety and that the operation poses some threat to their sexual identity as well as to that of the woman. Comments such as 'Well, you're no good . . . you can't have any more children' (Williams, 1972) indicate disapproval, lack of support and negative feelings to the woman and cause her to suffer anxiety and distress. Women have reported that they felt 'altered sexually' because of the different way they were treated by their partners after hysterectomy (Dennerstein *et al.*, 1977).

The circulation of these myths can lead to problems for women and those close to them, and knowledge of the facts about recovery from hysterectomy would help to break the cycle of perpetuation and reinforcement. Very real distress results, and is manifested by delayed or complicated recovery and dissatisfaction with the results of the operation.

Research on Recovery from Hysterectomy

Research on recovery from hysterectomy reports a variety of symptoms and problems which may be categorized as physical, psychological or sexual. Any classification such as this is obviously artificial because it may be difficult or impossible in real life to decide the source of problems. They are inter-related, and have feedback effects on one another. For example, a sexual problem may be a cause or effect of depression, or physical tiredness may lead to loss of libido and depression. Bearing this in mind, then, recovery will be described using these broad headings to structure the discussion.

Physical recovery

Weight gain is seen by many women as an almost inevitable consequence of hysterectomy, but researchers disagree about the extent and causes of this problem. Dalton (1957) explains the gain of one stone in weight by 50% of her patients within one year of operation as 'of the water retention type responding rapidly to fluid and salt restriction, diurectics and dieting'. She does not state whether her patients had had bilateral salpingo-oophorectomy as well as hysterectomy, and no hormone assays were done. It is not clear, therefore, why the patients should retain fluid or which of the treatments led to weight reduction. More recent research suggests that:

> 'Gain of weight after hysterectomy is generally due to sedentary habits in convalescence with no corresponding reduction in calorific intake. Anxiety associated with hysterectomy may precipitate increased eating.' (Dennerstein *et al.*, 1977)

Hot flushes as a sequel to hysterectomy have been widely reported, but, because many research samples include patients who have had both ovaries removed as well as those who have retained some functioning ovarian tissue, it is difficult to assess the extent of this problem. Masters and Johnson (1976) state that after hysterectomy the ovaries cease functioning sooner than they would otherwise, but no evidence of ovarian damage was found by Coppen *et al.* (1981). These workers used a variety of physiological measures to study 60 pre-menopausal women for up to three years after hysterectomy, and they conclude that there is no indication for giving oestrogen to these patients.

Urinary problems, especially frequency, seem to occur after hysterectomy. In Raphael's (1974) study in Australia of 100 married women under 46 years of age who had hysterectomy for non-malignant conditions, patients were categorized according to whether they had had a good or poor outcome on the basis of a mailed questionnaire sent 13 months after surgery. In the 'poor health' group, 52% of the women suffered from frequency of micturition. Comparison was also made with a control group from the general population and frequent urination occurred significantly more often ($p < 0.005$) in the hysterectomy patients. Cosper *et al.* (1978) found that 58% of their 40 subjects had difficulty in micturition in the first post-operative week but the number reduced to 23% five weeks after the operation. There is strong evidence, based on cytological and endoscopic tests, that for some post-hysterectomy patients, hormone deficiency, infection and obstruction due to post-operative scarring are causes of urinary problems (Smith *et al.*, 1970).

A variety of other physical symptoms has been reported during recovery from hysterectomy, including indigestion, constipation, backache, dizziness, headaches, sleep disturbances, and generalized aches and pains (Richards, 1974; Raphael, 1974). Richards attributes these to hormone deficiency. He found that insomnia was eight times more common in the hysterectomy patients he studied than in the control group of patients who had had other operations. Sleeplessness responded more readily to oral oestrogens than to hypnotics. Other workers, however, consider it more likely that these physical symptoms have psychosocial causes (Raphael, 1974; Dennerstein *et al.*, 1977).

Psychological recovery

Anxiety and depression related to threats to a woman's self-concept have been widely discussed in the literature, but research is often impaired by failure to use objective criteria to diagnose and measure disability.

A 'crisis of hysterectomy' is reported by Raphael (1972) on the basis of preliminary findings from a study of 100 hysterectomy patients and 100 controls who had undergone cholecystectomy. Sixty per cent of the hysterectomy patients experienced 'post-operative blues', with weeping, sadness and distress, usually four to five days after their operations. Only 20% of the cholecystectomy patients had this experience. Hysterectomy patients expressed dissatisfaction because their needs for emotional support had not been met, whereas control subjects felt these had been met. Raphael explains psychological distress after hysterectomy as being due to disappointment at lack of support and feeling of being let down by people whom patients expected to help them.

Aiming to determine the incidence of depressive symptoms 12 weeks after hysterectomy and to identify risk factors for the prediction of post-operative depression, Moore and Tolley (1976) used the Zung Self-Rating Scale as a measuring tool. Forty-seven women completed the scale the day before their operations, and again 12 weeks later. Thirty-two per cent were depressed when followed up, compared with 36% who had been depressed pre-operatively. The majority of the post-operative depressives existed prior to the operation. Other researchers also suggest that a history of psychiatric illness is associated with an increased risk of post-operative psychiatric symptoms, particularly depression (Richards, 1974; Polivy, 1974; Dennerstein *et al.*, 1977; Gath, 1980).

Sexual aspects of recovery

Once again the evidence is contradictory in relation to sexual activity after hysterectomy. Some women are anxious (Raphael, 1974), that the operation will mean 'the end of all sexual life, at least in a feeling way' (Hollender, 1960). Hysterectomy may, on the other hand, be seen as offering hope of improving long-standing psychosexual difficulties when all else has failed (Raphael, 1978).

Krueger *et al.* (1979) studied sexual adjustment to hysterectomy, and the effect of nurse counselling on this. A measure called 'sexual satisfaction following surgery' was formed by grouping three variables termed 'sexual pattern', 'enjoyment of sexual intercourse' and 'perception of partner's enjoyment of sexual intercourse'. Women who had more frequent sexual intercourse pre-operatively had more positive scores on this sexual satisfaction measure. Also, the younger the woman, the more likely she was to rate her sexual adjustment as positive. No significant relationship was found between sexual adjustment eight weeks post-operatively and nurse counselling about sexuality.

Masters and Johnson (1976) consider that after a medically necessary operation levels of interest in sex will improve in comparison with pre-operative levels. Loss of libido, when it occurs, is attributed to self-fulfilling prophecies of old wives' tales.

Positive support from sexual partners is an important influence on the recovery process and, conversely, negative attitudes and comments about the hysterectomy are detrimental. Some partners are more understanding in relation to sexual matters after the operation but others treat the woman differently and thereby convey negative impressions to her (Dennerstein *et al.*, 1977). Men may be indifferent to their partners' fears (Masters and Johnson, 1976), or may see hysterectomy as a reflection on their own sexual functioning and regard the woman as 'desexed' (Raphael, 1978). Raphael thinks that the partner is the person 'whose interest, concern and acceptance are paramount', and that his disapproval, lack of support or negative feelings about the operation are likely to lead to anxiety and distress for the woman.

Implications for future research

Research on recovery from hysterectomy is difficult to interpret and therefore firm conclusions cannot be drawn about the incidence of problems and measures to prevent or treat them. The reason for this is that in many cases a mixed sample is used which includes patients having had a simple hysterectomy as well as those also having had bilateral salpingo-oophorectomy. Some reports categorize together women undergoing surgery for benign and malignant conditions. It is then impossible to separate the different effects of a major operation which can threaten the self-concept from those of a surgically induced menopause or fears of cancer.

Self-concept seems to be an important factor, however, and methodologically sound research is needed to look in more detail at its influence on recovery. It might then be possible to see how to help women and their partners to adjust more smoothly to the major life event of hysterectomy.

Past research can give some guidelines for future studies by identifying variables which may be important in influencing the effect on self-concept. Personality disposition may be important in adjustment to hysterectomy, just as it has been shown to be in other cases (Polivy, 1974; Wilson-Barnett, 1978). Anxious women may be more likely to view this operation as threatening, and younger patients may be more affected by the loss of their reproductive functions (Raphael, 1974; Moore and Tolley, 1976). Those women who have not had children or who would have liked to add to their families may be more likely to regret having the operation because they see themselves as having failed as a woman. Child-bearing is differentially valued according to social class and culture, and if femininity is defined in these terms, women may be more distressed by hysterectomy because it affects how significant others value and support them (Raphael, 1978; Williams, 1972).

Promotion of Good Recovery from Hysterectomy

If more was known about which factors interfered with or promoted adjustment after hysterectomy it might be possible to take preventive measures before problems had a chance to occur.

Pre-operative screening is advocated by some workers to evaluate the need for surgery, detect 'at risk' patients and pick up possible warnings that complications may develop later. Screening should focus on 'careful searching out and dispellation of myths and groundless fears' (Polivy, 1974). Pre-existing depression or other emotional disturbances should be diagnosed and treated before surgery to try to minimize later recurrences (Green, 1973; Thompson, 1975; Moore and Tolley, 1976).

Giving information to patients so that they know what to expect of the operation and its effects is advocated by many surgeons and nurses. Some emphasize the need to include the sexual partner because he can have such a profound influence on the woman's self-concept (Raphael, 1978; Dennerstein *et al.*, 1977). Patients should know the nature of the operation, the reasons for it, and its expected effects, and a simple diagram should be used to aid the explanation (Dennerstein *et al.*, 1977). General instructions to 'take it easy' are not specific enough. Women want more concrete advice on which activities are difficult and should be delayed (Williams, 1976; Cosper *et al.*, 1978). The same applies to sexual activity—women need to know what effects to expect, what not to expect and when they may resume sexual intercourse. They should be warned about the possibility of certain symptoms occurring during convalescence and told what action to take in these circumstances. All this information should be accompanied by an explanation of the reasons, and counselling should be carried out in a way which gives the patient opportunities to ask for additional advice and to discuss aspects she may not fully understand (Raphael, 1978). Williams (1978) concludes that 'nurses can contribute importantly to women's post-hysterectomy recovery by being sensitive to individual feelings, by telling patients what to expect and why, and by exploring with them their questions and ideas about the effects of hysterectomy'. A leaflet which incorporates these recommendations has been designed by Steele and Goodwin (1975) who advocate its use to reinforce a verbal explanation.

An on-going study of recovery from hysterectomy is being carried out by the author of this section of the chapter (and J.W.-B.). Its aims are to describe recovery in order to clarify some of the contradictions noted in previous research, and to test the effect on recovery of an experimental counselling session. The sample size of 150 patients should permit reliable conclusions to be drawn, and only patients having simple hysterectomy are included; that is, subjects must be having the operation for benign conditions and must retain some ovarian function.

The study has a cross-over design which involves two researchers, both experienced gynaecological ward sisters. Patients are interviewed by researcher A on their fifth or sixth post-operative day. Personal information is collected, together with details of the patient's previous medical history and her feelings about having the operation. In addition, they complete the Eysenck Personality Inventory (Eysenck and Eysenck, 1964), a Mood Adjective Check-List (McNair and Lorr, 1964), the Beck Depression Inventory (Beck *et al.*, 1961) and a Self-Concept Scale based on that developed by Pearlin and Schooler (1978). Researcher B visits the hospital the following day, randomly allocates patients to one of three experimental groups, and conducts the counselling session. Patients assigned to the control group receive no contact at this stage. Those in the experimental groups are counselled about the operation and their recovery, while those in the placebo group have a conversation of equal length about general topics and avoiding the subject of the operation and recovery. Researcher A, who is unaware of the group to which the patient is allocated, visits the patients in their homes four months after the operation to conduct an extensive interview focussing on experiences and feelings during recovery, and the psychological tests are repeated. The two researchers change roles every 15 patients.

The experimental counselling aims to explain the hysterectomy and its effects, guide patients in controlling their own recovery, tell them of minor symptoms which may occur as part of the recovery process and how to deal with them, and to give women a chance to ventilate their feelings about having a hysterectomy. A simple diagram is shown, and the researcher indicates which organs have been removed and which remain intact and functioning, emphasizing that the patient will not begin the 'change of life' and that her ability to have sexual intercourse, her sexual attractiveness and feelings should not change as a result of the operation. She is told that every woman is an individual and therefore will have a unique recovery experience. She will be able to control her progress by using her own feelings and tiredness as guides to how much to do and when to avoid over-strenuous activities. Symptoms such as weight gain, constipation, backache, wound discomfort, vaginal bleeding and tearfulness are mentioned, together with an explanation of why they may occur and how to deal with them. For example, weight gain is said not to be a direct consequence of the specific surgery but to be caused by inactivity and/or overeating during convalescence, and so it can be controlled by diet as at any other time.

This research will be completed by the end of 1982 and should give a full picture of how women are likely to progress after hysterectomy and how nurses can help their patients to recover as smoothly and completely as possible. It should show the extent to which women's self-concept is affected by the operation and indicate which factors are important in meeting and counteracting this threat.

Increasing attention was given in the literature on hysterectomy in the 1960's and 1970's on the interplay between self-concept and cultural beliefs and attitudes regarding the female role. This parallels changing social definitions of femininity and the sexual division of labour in our own culture. There has been speculation that, as these changes become more widespread, attitudes towards hysterectomy will also change and its emotional consequences will be less traumatic for women's self-concept (Masters and Johnson, 1976; Notman, 1976; Derogatis, 1980). In this developing situation it is essential for nurses and doctors to be aware that hysterectomy can have major implications for their patients' self-concept, and to take responsibility for preparing women comprehensively for their recovery.

References

Beck, A. T., Ward, G. H., Mendelson, M., Mock, J., and Erbaugh, J. (1961). An inventory for measuring depression. *Archives of General Psychiatry,* **4**, 561–571.

Coppen, A., Bishop, M., Beard, R. J., Barnard, G. J. R., and Collins, W. P. (1981). Hysterectomy, hormones and behaviour. *Lancet,* **i**, 126–128.

Cosper, B., Fuller, S. S., and Robinson, G. J. (1978). Characteristics of post-hospitalisation recovery following hysterectomy. *Journal of Obstetric and Gynaecological Nursing,* **7**, 7–11.

Dalton, K. (1957). Discussion on the aftermath of hysterectomy and oophorectomy. *Proceedings of the Royal Society of Medicine, Section of General Practice,* **50**, 415–418.

Dennerstein, L., Wood, G., and Burrows, G. (1977). Sexual dysfunction following hysterectomy. *Australian Family Physician,* **6**, 535–543.

Derogatis, L. R. (1980). Breast and gynaecologic cancers: their unique impact on body image and sexual identity in women. In J. M. Vaeth (Editor), *Frontiers of Radiation Therapy and Oncology,* Vol.14. Karger, Basel, pp. 1–11.

Eysenck, H. J., and Eysenck, S. B. G. (1964). *Manual of the Eysenck Personality Inventory.* University of London Press, London.

Garrity, T. F., Somes, G. W., and Marx, M. B. (1977). Personality factors in resistance to illness after recent life changes. *Journal of Psychosomatic Research,* **21**, 23–32.

Gath, D. (1980). Psychiatric aspect of hysterectomy. In L. Robins, P. Clayton and J. Wing (Editors), *The Social Consequences of Psychiatric Illness.* Brunner/Mazel Inc., New York.

Gore, S. (1978). The effect of social support in moderating the health consequences of unemployment. *Journal of Health and Social Behaviour,* **19**, 157–165.

Green, R. L. (1973). The emotional aspects of hysterectomy. *Southern Medical Journal,* **66**, 442–444.

Hollender, M. H. (1960). A study of patients admitted to psychiatric hospital after pelvic operations. *American Journal of Obstetrics and Gynecology,* **79**, 498–503.

Krueger, J. C. (1979). Relationship between nurse counselling and sexual adjustment after hysterectomy. *Nursing Research,* **3**, 145–150.

Masters, W. H., and Johnson, V. (1976). What young women should know about hysterectomies. *Redbook,* Jan., 48–51.

McNair, D. M., and Lorr, M. (1964). An analysis of mood in neurotics. *Journal of Abnormal and Social Psychology,* **69**, 620–627.

Moore, J. T., and Tolley, D. H. (1976). Depression following hysterectomy. *Psychosomatics,* **17**, 86–89.

Notman, M. T. (1976). Elective hysterectomy: pro and con. *New England Journal of Medicine,* **295**, 5 266–267.

Pearlin, I. C., and Schooler, C. (1978). The structure of coping. *Journal of Health and Social Behaviour,* **19**, 2–21.

Polivy, J. (1974). Psychological reactions to hysterectomy: a critical review. *Journal of Obstetrics and Gynaecology,* **118**, 417–426.

Raphael, B. (1972). The crisis of hysterectomy. *Australian and New Zealand Journal of Psychiatry,* **6**, 106–115.

Raphael, B. (1974). Parameters of health outcome following hysterectomy. *Bulletin of Post-graduate Committee in Medicine,* University of Sydney, Dec., 214–219.

Raphael, B. (1978). Psychiatric aspects of hysterectomy. In J. G. Howells (Editor), *Modern Perspectives in the Psychiatric Aspects of Surgery.* Macmillan, London.

Richards, D. H. (1974). A post-hysterectomy syndrome. *Lancet,* **ii**, 983–985.

Rosenberg, M. (1965). *Society and the Adolescent Self-image.* Princeton University Press, New Jersey.

Smith, P., Roberts, M., and Slade, N. (1970). Urinary symptoms following hysterectomy. *British Journal of Urology,* **42**, 3–9.

Steele, S. J., and Goodwin, M. R. (1975). A pamphlet to answer the patients' questions before hysterectomy. *Lancet,* **ii**, 492–493.

Thompson, V. M. (1975). Sexual life after hysterectomy. *British Medical Journal*, **iii**, 304.

Williams, M. A. (1972). A comparative study of post-surgical convalescence among women of 2 ethnic groups: Anglo and Mexican-American. *Community Nursing Research,* **5**, Nov., 59–73.

Williams, M. A. (1976). Easier convalescence after hysterectomy. *American Journal of Nursing,* **76**, 3, 438–440.

Wilson-Barnett, J. (1978). Patients emotional reactions to barium X-rays. *Journal of Advanced Nursing,* **3**, 37–45.

Wolf, S. R. (1970). Emotional reactions to hysterectomy. *Postgraduate Medical Journal,* **47**, 165–169.

CHAPTER 5

Recovery from Ischaemic Heart Disease

Diseases of the heart may be seen as particularly stressful. Patients have to adjust to a potentially life-threatening condition and sometimes to surgery which has a relatively high mortality rate. Because of the seriousness of ischaemic heart disease and the mental strain for the patient, it is not surprising that recovery from a myocardial infarction is often complicated by psychological problems. Recovery in this area has been assessed in various ways, from the mortality and morbidity rates used in clinical studies to the degree of social recovery and return to work, attempting to assess the quality of life. In this chapter, problems of recovery after heart attack will be reviewed with studies evaluating ways to avoid them. The outcome of surgery, grafting coronary arteries, will then be discussed with details of a recently completed study by the author (J.W.-B.).

RECOVERY FROM HEART ATTACK

Many studies have documented that patients feel extremely anxious when admitted to a coronary care unit with chest pain and suspected infarction. For instance, Cay *et al.* (1972) examined patients in the unit and found that 30% of patients were severely upset after their first infarct and 42% were after a subsequent attack. More recently, Lloyd and Cawley (1978) found 35% of their sample of 100 consecutive admissions to have psychiatric morbidity. Specialists in the psychological care of these patients such as Degree-Coustry (1976) consider that the severity of early emotional responses influences subsequent recovery. Characteristic responses range from 'panic, fear of death, a feeling of handicap and impotence'.

Currently, 'heart attack' patients have a gentle mobilization programme over ten days in hospital, if their early care in the coronary care unit has been uncomplicated. This avoids the prolonged period of enforced dependence which was so debilitating. However, reports from a decade ago by Wynn (1967) give evidence of poor communications in the ward and lack of necessary support and information for patients, which is echoed in more recent work, reviewed below. Wynn considered that poor recovery at home—50% of such patients becoming cardiac invalids, disabled by neurosis—was a direct consequence of overprotection during hospitalization and lack of guidance for patients after discharge from hospital.

Although recently patients are apparently less obviously crippled by a heart attack, recovery is often complicated by psychological problems; for instance, Mayou *et al.* (1978a), studying 100 patients one year after infarction, found substantial psychological distress resulting from changes in social activities and relationships, for both patients and their families. Although 60% of patients had returned to work within 12 weeks of the onset of their illness, many problems over other aspects of life were prevalent. The authors discuss the many adjustments made by patients and their families in regard to their level of activity at work and leisure. Thirty per cent of patients had made major changes in leisure activities and 36% had made smaller changes. Seventy per cent reported they were quite satisfied with their leisure although about a third of the sample had reduced their social outings to some extent. Just over half these patients had returned to more or less the same pattern as their previous lifestyle by the end of the year. With respect to relationships, a quarter of the sample noted a positive improvement in their marriage, a half noticed no change and the remainder reported deterioration, conflict and tension. Family life tended to be affected to the same degree. Obviously other stresses and life events had a compounding effect on ease of rehabilitation.

In this study of rehabilitation by Mayou *et al.* (1978a) outcome measures were assessed, scored and totalled. Twenty-four patients had a positive outcome with the 'same' or 'better' than previous activity and interaction patterns. Of the remainder, 32 patients had the greatest deterioration in their social life. Poor rehabilitation was associated in part with severe physical problems and poor pre-morbid personalities. A small group could be identified as having done badly or well in all areas, but for the majority of patients there was no single aspect of outcome which determined measures of rehabilitation. In conclusion to this work, the authors state, 'Whilst for many patients outcome is satisfactory, psychological and social morbidity is significant.' Return to work is seen as a priority for patients, but most of them reduced their level of activity in leisure, social contacts and sexual relations, which tended to reduce their satisfaction with life as a whole. Satisfactory rehabilitation was said to be influenced by a stable pre-morbid personality, few additional life events and a supportive home environment.

The role of the family and spouse's (usually the wife) support is frequently seen as a vital factor in promoting a full rehabilitation, but this is made very difficult when they are not given enough information to provide support and encouragement. In an earlier study by Mayou *et al.* (1976) with 40 patients and their relatives, the most common problem was couples' low degree of understanding of medical advice and information. Despite great satisfaction with treatment, communications were seen as 'inadequate, vague and conflicting'. Patients saw the doctor as the main information giver but did not like to ask about treatment or admitted that they did not know what they needed to be told. Relatives saw much less of the doctors or nursing staff than the patients and expressed uncertainty about the seriousness and consequences of the infarct. They found the hospital environment very alarming and were diffident about approaching the doctor to ask for guidance at home. General practitioners were seen to be more approachable although their advice was often rather vague and unhelpful. The out-patient follow-up visit was again disappointing from this point of view—a long wait was usually followed by a rushed consultation.

The authors discuss these findings in relation to a lack of coordinated policies for information giving and grave lack of awareness of patients' needs on the part of staff, many of whom, particularly junior doctors, were unsure about what advice to give patients. The event of returning home often confronts the patient with so many more problems than have been unexpected. They recommend that nurses could supervise and coordinate convalescence.

The importance of including wives in any counselling sessions is evidenced by further work of Mayou's team (1978b). Eighty-two wives were interviewed while their husbands were in hospital, two months after their discharge and again one year after they went home. Psychological symptoms were noted at two months, and also at one year they were still considerable. Forty per cent complained of ill health themselves during this year. Wives were anxious to care for their husbands correctly yet lacked clear advice as to when they could lift, how far they could walk, etc. They were still active in helping the patient to convalesce a year after discharge, frequently consulting the GP, administering tablets and diet.

However, a third were still over-protective. The wives who were least distressed at one year were those who continued to work themselves and had independent leisure activities. Wives' adjustment was related to both their earlier mental state and their husband's mental state at one year. It was not related to the husband's physical state, economic burdens or restricted social life. They concluded for this study that wives' psychological disability was often more severe than that of the patient at the initial onset of illness but throughout the year 'was considerable, persistent and comparable to that of the patients themselves'.

In the light of problems in the recovery of coronary patients it is relevant to look at specific risk factors. The comprehensive clinical and interview three-stage follow-up study by Croog and Levine (1977) assessed factors which influenced recovery one year after a heart attack for 293 patients. They found that family and social support had an essential positive relationship with good recovery, whereas re-admission to hospital had a major negative influence. Surprisingly, patients' self-perception and the severity of their infarction was independent of recovery. Return to work, an event associated with economic, social and personal factors, was influenced more by occupational and employment opportunities than patients' motivation. Blue collar workers remained the unemployed casualities, which was considered totally unnecessary in terms of their physical capacity after exercise training.

Croog and Levine (1977) also found that physicians were able to predict recovery from the patient's history and family situation quite well. Criteria used for assessment during this first year were major illness with hospitalization, associated disease, other diseases, return to work, level of compliance, patient's rating of their outcome, satisfaction levels, mood ratings and maintenance of pre-illness levels of activity. Their contribution to research in this area is substantial, as only a decade before they acknowledged the great difficulty of measurement and comparison in rehabilitation (Croog *et al.*, 1968) in one of the first reviews across many specialities.

With knowledge of morbidity and risk factors, staff should be attempting to improve the situation. In an extremely comprehensive review of the effect of exercise on patients after infarction, Shephard (1981) has concluded that graduated exercise programmes hold no additional risk factors but that they may give good psychological benefit. Although there are few experimentally controlled studies it appears that counselling in re-employment and for general worries does help prevent psychological problems. For example, employment abilities and opportunities were shown to be significantly increased by a positive approach with a multidisciplinary team in Schillar and Baker's (1976) controlled trial with two groups of over 100 patients. Return to work is therefore less dependent on physical recovery or personal drive than many assume. Predictive factors for returning to employment were listed as: previous employment prior to hospitalization, stability of patient's work history, patient's opinion that a job was available after his recovery, family and social stability, age of starting smoking, personality predisposition to anxiety and depression, educational level, types of previous work. These and other researchers advise more active involvement by professionals in supporting and helping patients gain the confidence to return to work.

Another, more recent, controlled study by Naismith *et al.* (1979) assessed the effect of a nurse giving psychological counselling after myocardial infarction for patients and their wives. This demonstrated how effective planned and repeated support sessions and guidance from a nurse could be for recovery. A significant improvement on return to work, physical and emotional stability and social independence was found for the experimental group, each of these three categories being measured on a simple three-point scale rated by the research team. Positive or negative attitude towards recovery was influential and those patients with a high neuroticism score had a slower recovery but were responsive to extra counselling. This study, as well as others evaluating intervention, may reflect patients' appreciation and gratitude for professional attention. This in itself was thought by Graham *et al.* (1979) to be of major benefit in recovery from a heart attack.

In an experiment with three groups of post-myocardial infarction patients, Mayou *et al.* (1981) compared the effects of eight exercise sessions (two each week) with three or four advisory sessions and with usual after-care. Their results confirm previous studies that exercise did not affect cardiac function in the long term but it gave patients confidence to be more active throughout their recovery, despite more psychological symptoms than others. Counselling, on the other hand, prevented over-protective attitudes from patients' families and resulted in more patients being pleased with their overall outcome. There was a comparatively low overall rate (11%) of psychological complications in this sample of 129 patients. Exercise patients were more satisfied with their rehabilitation sessions than those receiving advice sessions. There was a 24% non-attendance overall and of these patients tended not to regard themselves 'back to normal' at three months, in contrast to 46% of the attenders. Mayou's team recommend planned and individualized rehabilitation sessions, particularly for the highly anxious patients, but recognize that those most in need often fall into the non-attending group.

As early as 1959, Hellerstein was encouraging careful study of individual patient's work history and performance in laboratory stress tests to assess their capacity and provide clearer guides as to what levels were required for different jobs. However, there is still a need for a carefully designed and generally applicable inventory of work-activity competence to assess patients' real potential for returning to work. As Wintner and Kellerman (1976) state, this is essential for encouraging those who find difficulties in this area.

Conclusions from a review on patient experiences after an infarction (Wilson-Barnett, 1979) still apply:

(1) Anxiety is the most common initial response to myocardial infarction. For the majority of patients it is their condition rather than the coronary care unit which evokes this response. Denial of the severity of this condition is frequently seen as a defence against this anxiety.
(2) Over-cautious staff who encourage lengthy periods of bedrest and dependence are said to encourage over-anxious patients.
(3) Severe anxiety and depression are frequently experienced by patients during the post-infarct year.
(4) When return to work is delayed or postponed indefinitely, emotional problems are as frequently the cause of, or more so than, physical complications.
(5) Although as many as four out of five patients return to work, there are grave problems of adjustment in social and leisure activity for 30%.
(6) Lack of systematic support and information giving throughout treatment is frequently blamed for many of the emotional rehabilitation problems.
(7) Support for the spouse, or close relative, is also needed and clear guidelines for rehabilitation activities should be given to the patient and their family.
(8) There is now evidence that fairly rapid mobilization is indicated for uncomplicated myocardial infarction patients.
(9) Nurses are said to have a potentially important role in initiating and maintaining programmes for psychological and physical rehabilitation.

Planned teaching of patients and preparing both partners for recovery at home is rarely carried out (see Wilson-Barnett, 1981) despite evidence that it gives patients more knowledge (Bracken *et al.*, 1977) and that aspects related to home life are particularly relevant and important for patients (Rahe *et al.*, 1975). Because of the serious problems encountered by patients, staff should become more involved in giving psychological care and guidance for recovery. It is important to be optimistic about a patient's prognosis. An uncomplicated recovery bodes well for the majority, and a well-balanced plan for moderate exercise, weight reduction, reducing stress and cessation of smoking can give many years of good living. Despite the many very detailed guidelines for rehabilitation, Shephard (1981) found that no significant factors were of particular benefit. It is therefore wise for patients to learn to relax, and build up exercise tolerance gradually. Above all, careless remarks about their limitations by staff and family should be castigated. Most of the care needed for these patients is psychological—their fears being the main source of impaired recovery. This group demonstrates how hospitalization can so easily delay recovery.

References

Bracken, M. B., Bracken, M., and Landry, A. B. (1977). Patient education by videotape after myocardial infarction: An empirical evaluation 1967. *Archives of Physical Medicine and Rehabilitation,* **58**, 213–219.

Cay, E. L., Vetter, N., Philips, A. E., and Digard, P. (1972). Psychological status during recovery from an acute heart attack. *Journal of Psychosomatic Research,* **16**, 425–435.

Croog, S. H., and Levine, S. (1977). *The Heart Patient Recovers.* Human Science Press, New York.

Croog, S. H., Levine, S., and Lurie, Z. (1968). The heart patient and the recovery process. A review of the directions of research on social and psychological factors. *Social Science and Medicine,* **2**, 111–164.

Degree-Coustry, C. (1976). Psychological problems in rehabilitation programmes. In V. Stocksmeier, (Editor), *Psychological Approach to the Rehabilitation of Coronary Patients.* Springer-Verlag, New York.

Graham, I., Mulcaty, R., and Hickey, N. (1979). Correspondence. *British Medical Journal*, **i**, 549.

Hellerstein, H. K. (1959). Intereducation and re-education in the rehabilitation of the cardiac patient. *American Heart Journal*, **58**, 425–435.

Lloyd, G. G., and Cawley, R. H. (1978). Psychiatric morbidity in men one week after first myocardial infarction. *British Medical Journal*, **ii**, 1453–1454.

Mayou, R., Williamson, B., and Foster, A. (1976). Attitudes and advice after myocardial infarction. *British Medical Journal*, **i**, 1577–1579.

Mayou, R., Foster, A., and Williamson, B. (1978a). Psychosocial adjustment in patients one year after myocardial infarction. *Journal of Psychosomatic Research,* **22**, 447–453.

Mayou, R., Foster, A., and Williamson, B. (1978b). The psychological and social effects of myocardial infarction on wives. *British Medical Journal,* **i**, 699–701.

Mayou, R., MacMahon, D., Sleight, P., and Florence, M. T. (1981). Early rehabilitation after myocardial infarction. *Lancet,* **ii**, 1399–1401.

Naismith, L. D., Robinson, J. F., Shaw, G. B., and MacIntyre, M. M. J. (1979). Psychological rehabilitation after myocardial infarction. *British Medical Journal,* **i**, 439–446.

Rahe, R. H., Scalzi, C., and Shine, K. (1975). A teaching evaluation questionnaire for post myocardial infarction patients. *Heart and Lung,* **4**, 759–766.

Schillar, E., and Baker, J. (1976). Return to work after a myocardial infarction evaluation of planned rehabilitation and of a predictive rating scale. *Medical Journal of Australia,* **i**, 859–862.

Shephard, R. J. (1981). *Ischaemic Heart Disease and Exercise.* Croom Helm, London.

Wilson-Barnett, J. (1979). A review of research into the experience of patients suffering from coronary thrombosis. *International Journal of Nursing Studies,* **16**, 183–198.

Wilson-Barnett, J. (1981). Patient teaching—after myocardial infarction. *Nursing,* **38**, 1398–1399.

Wintner, I., and Kellermann, J. J. (1976). Psychological factors involved in cardiac rehabilitation. In V. Stocksmeier (Editor), *Psychological Approach to the Rehabilitation of Coronary Patients.* Springer-Verlag, New York.

Wynn, A. (1967). Unwarranted emotional distress in men with ischaemic heart disease (IHD). *Medical Journal of Australia,* **ii**, 847–851.

RECOVERY FROM SURGERY FOR ISCHAEMIC HEART DISEASE

Since the first exploratory operation transplanting the saphenous vein to the coronary arteries in 1964, over 300 000 operations have been performed (for instance, 1500 operations were done in 1975 in Great Britain), but 'only 1248 (series) have been reported which have been studied in a carefully controlled and random manner' (McIntosh and Garcia, 1978). It is now established (Editorial, *Lancet*, 1979) that this is more effective for pain relief than medication in most cases, but there are reservations for claims by Lawrie *et al.* (1978) and the European Coronary Surgery Study Group (1980) that surgery prolongs life or prevents mortality from myocardial infarctions. Risk factors are also well established (Mundth and Austen, 1975).

Studies are now less devoted to evaluating morbidity and mortality but are more concerned in assessing the level of recovery in the longer term, once more tending to concentrate on return to work. Excellent reviews of such studies exist by McIntosh and Garcia (1978) and Preston (1977). Both criticize the lack of prospective, truly random controlled studies and the lack of defined criteria by which to judge the quality of life and health post-operatively. Preston is particularly sceptical about the assessments using pain ratings, where surgeons may influence patients' reports and where the operation has been shown to reduce pain even when grafts no longer remain patent. Lack of longer-term assessments for many years has also masked the evidence that coronary artery disease may be accelerated in post-operative patients.

Studies that attempt to evaluate social outcome are far outnumbered by those clinical follow-up studies which attempt to identify risk factors, to demonstrate low mortality and morbidity rates for their series, or to prove that surgical therapy is more effective for pain relief and longevity. This larger group use common physical criteria listed below and usually rely on clinical records for data. Where social aspects (return to work) are considered these are not compared with general population norms. A huge range has been reported. Rimm *et al.* (1976), in a five-year clinical follow-up study at two large American centres with 893 men, found failure to return to work as low as 11% in younger men and 26% in the older age range. In Britain, a smaller study of 115 patients by Wallwork *et al.* (1978), using interviews and questionnaires, found 75 patients returning to work, 59 of these within two to six months post-operatively. Other studies have been less positive in their results, such as those of Barnes' team (1975), where there was an overall loss to the work force in hours as compared to the pre-operative situation. Oberman and Kouchoukos (1979) concluded from their review that the main predictor of not returning to work was the length of time off work pre-operatively. They discussed how habit formation and adjustment to unemployment as well as the social rewards of this situation, of help from others and visitors to the home, and to increased financial gains from social security benefits were also shown to discourage attempts to find work. Overall the economic rationalization for maintaining an expensive cardiac surgery programme has certainly encouraged the protestant ethic of 'working status' to be used for this group of patients. It is limited by economic and social opportunities and the age of retirement of many of these patients. The results are conflicting, and this criterion should have been compared with other indications of benefit from surgery.

Other studies have approached recovery from the psychological or psychiatric perspective. For instance, Pilowsky *et al.* (1979) studied attitudes prior to surgery in order to assess their relationship to outcome, in particular relief from angina. In this prospective research the 'Illness Behaviour Questionnaire' was completed by 122 patients before surgery. Good recovery was associated with a high responsiveness to reassurance, low inter-personal discord, high illness vulnerability, low pain-related-illness anxiety, low irritability and low health concern. These dimensions may be related to low general emotionality and good adjustment and possibly use of denial. A good outcome was noted in three-quarters of the sample.

In an uncharacteristic study for this group of patients, using psychiatric interview, Gundle *et al.* (1980) monitored psychosocial recovery in 30 post-operative patients, one to two years after coronary bypass surgery. They state, 'investigators have given little attention to psychological and social outcome.' With their sample they noted that 69% reached maximum practical exercise tolerance, but despite this good outcome 83% were unemployed and 57% were impotent. Other manifestations of maladjustment included restricted social life, low self-esteem and lack of pleasure in social life. 'A small but significant number of patients revealed persistent dependency needs of varying severity, serious distortions of body image and symptomatic depression.' They explain these problems in part by the long pre-operative experience of angina and the persistent 'damage' to the self-image. It is obviously difficult to discuss these findings in the light of unquantified data from such a small number of patients. However, there is other evidence that predisposition to psychiatric problems would certainly influence post-operative outcome. With a sample of 100 patients Willner and Rabiner (1979) found that those with psychopathology were more likely to die post-operatively. One fifth of these patients had psychiatric symptoms during the five years after surgery. Once more it is difficult to gain a perspective on the gravity of this situation from the published material.

Researchers are now attempting to assess the quality of life after surgery and to discuss the difficulty of measuring this nebulous but essential outcome criterion. However, most of the content of results is still directed to reinstatement in employment or household activities. For instance, Mendola and Pelligrini (1979) discuss that more meaningful measures are needed to evaluate a patient's social situation and physical capacity as well as the patient's satisfaction. They define quality of life as 'the individual's achievement of a satisfactory social situation within the limits of perceived physical capacity.' Patients were asked whether they had limits to what they could do. This was assessed at one structured interview, between six months and three years post-operatively, for 95 patients. Sixty per cent had no physical limitation and this reflects the patients' high overall satisfaction. Only 12% who wished to work were still unemployed and levels of activity were said to be related to whether patients perceived that physical activity or rest had helped most during their recovery.

The overall success of pain relief, return to work and small levels of mortality from surgery now seem generalized. Of recent British studies this is reflected in a retrospective study by Westaby *et al.* (1979) where 90% of their sample of patients returned to work; this included two-thirds of the manual workers. Quality of life was assessed by questionnaire in terms of resuming hobbies (70.8%), gardening (68.7%), social activities (76.9%) and sexual intercourse (71.8%). Likewise, in a study of 'the quality of life after cardiac surgery for valvular and artery disease', Ross *et al.* (1981) in a five-stage interview study with 383 patients (only 39 of whom had arterial grafts) used ability to leave house unaccompanied, physical independence and lack of limitation on activity as the main criteria for 'quality' measurement. Certainly leisure activities and reports of improvement in mood were also mentioned.

Given the difficulties in gaining data on criteria which are universally applicable to the sample, it may not be surprising that the methods used have relied on such broad topics. However, it appears that cardiac

Table 4 Criteria used to evaluate outcome and recovery

	Frequency of use*
Mortality rate—length of survival	F
Morbidity—serious complication	F
Physical condition by exercise testing	F
cardiac function	F
angiography	F
Patency of grafts	F
Symptoms—pain	F
dyspnoea	F
Return to work	F
Activity levels (other than work)	R
Compliance with medical advice	R
Social activity, hobbies	R
Financial status	R
Sexual activity	R
Satisfaction with operation	R
Family response	E
Psychological status—affect	E
adjustment	E
self-esteem	E
perception of health status	E
Resumption of normal life	E
'Minor' problems	E
Satisfaction with advice and guidance	E
Patient's understanding of treatment	E

*F = frequently, R = rarely, E = exceptionally.

specialists concentrate on the favourable and more global aspects of outcome usually assessed at out-patient follow-up visits, and where others interview patients there is a greater possibility that more detail in reporting would reveal very different information. It is also interesting that only one article discussed 'minor' complications such as pain from the sternotomy or swelling of the leg after removal of the vein (Logue *et al.*, 1976).

A list of the criteria used in studies of outcome is given in Table 4, and the indication is that more social and psychological measures are needed. Preston (1977) urges the use of better evaluative methods, stating that,

> 'Improved methodology is possible through the use of:
> (a) Standardised questions designed to elicit the level of activity by the patient.
> (b) Interviewers not associated by the patient as part of the medical process (interviewers could be trained health personnel in non-medical dress and in non-medical setting).
> (c) Confidential interviews with persons who know the patient well.'

The Follow-up Study

It therefore seemed appropriate that when a British cardiac team wished to monitor their progress they asked a nurse to interview patients. Post-operative coronary artery graft (CABG) patients were interviewed one year after surgery in the out-patients' department. Specifically this aimed to:

(1) obtain information on recovery from this surgery, from the patient's perspective;
(2) assess psychological and physical problems during recovery;
(3) calculate the range of time necessary for complete recovery;
(4) examine the needs for advice and guidance;
(5) assess whether dimensions of 'self-concept' were related to the degree of recovery.

Sample and methods

This study involved interviewing consecutive CABG patients attending the out-patients' department of one hospital for their annual post-operative visit. A letter was sent to each of these patients two weeks prior to their appointment, explaining the purpose of the study and asking for their help. This interview contained mostly open questions, four analogue and one linear scale and two psychological tests. Of these, one was a mood adjective check-list assessing levels of anxiety, depression, hostility, vigour and fatigue in the year since surgery (see Wilson-Barnett, 1977) and the second was a fifteen-item self-concept scale, modified and tested by Porritt (1979).

Sixty patients were interviewed over a 24-month period. Thirteen patients failed to attend or were unavoidably missed by the researcher. As with other studies the majority were male (55) and 10% were female (5). Only four of the patients lived alone, all were men. The average age of these patients was 57.4 years but there was a wide range (34–78 years). There was a normal socioeconomic distribution. Forty-four patients were in full-time employment (although usually interrupted by illness) prior to surgery, eight in heavy manual labouring. Ten patients had given up work prior to surgery, through illness; only six were already retired, this included one woman.

The number of arteries grafted per patient was as follows: 5 arteries for 2 patients, 4 for 25, 3 for 28, 2 for 3, and 1 for 2.

Results

Patients were classified according to their own reports on the extent of their recovery, as shown in Table 5. 35 (Group 1) were fully recovered,

Table 5 Recovery as reported by patients
(at least three responses fell in the same classification for all patients)

Questions	Group 1 $n=35$ Average age 57.8 years	Group 2 $n=19$ Average age 56.4 years	Group 3 $n=6$ Average age 58.5 years
What percentage would you give your present state of health?	> 80%	50–79%	< 49%
Has life returned to normal?	Yes	No	No
How has your recovery been, related to your expectations?	'Better' or 'As good as'	'Not quite so good'	'Worse than I expected'
Can you do all your usual activities?	Yes, no limitations	Most, slight limitations	No, severe limitations

reported resuming all activities they wished to do and had no emotional problems. At the other extreme, the six patients in Group 3 had considerable debility—two from severe infection in the sternal wound, three with persistent angina and depression, one with severe hypertension and slight senility from a past stroke. However, three of these patients said that they were better since the operation. The other 19 patients in Group 2 complained of leg and sternal pain, tiredness or recurrent, but rarely severe, angina. There were no overall differences in the ages of patients in these three groups. Two of the women were classified in Group 1 and three in Group 2.

Period of recovery

Recovery was also assessed by resumption of functions and whether the patients felt recovered. The range of time needed for full recovery, as perceived by the patients, ranged from two months to over a year. Thirty patients (27 were in Group 1) said that at two months they were feeling well and could do most things that they wished to. The majority (12) in Group 2 took longer to feel recovered ('on the whole'), on average about six months; the remainder still had health problems which prevented them feeling recovered (even 'on the whole'). However, at the yearly interview just under a third of the total sample from Groups 1 and 2 said they were recovered but were still improving!

At two months all patients had walked outside, 41 out of 46 could do their gardening (or equivalent exercises) and the same number had recommenced driving. Only 35 had resumed lifting what they considered a heavy weight (such as a car tyre or large packed suitcase) at two months. At one year, five patients had not resumed driving (three using the operation as a convenient event for giving up driving) and 25 patients did not consider lifting heavy weights, whether or not they could do it without symptoms (see Figure 4).

Early physical difficulties in the recovery period

Patients' lifestyle on return home was related to the availability of a spouse or friend who cared for them. Those who returned to live alone reported independence immediately, except for shopping done by a friend. For those who received help, the majority received domestic help, such as cooking and laundry. Twenty-one patients needed more personal help with bathing or dressing or sitting up in bed. Fifteen patients mentioned the problem of getting comfortable in bed and often

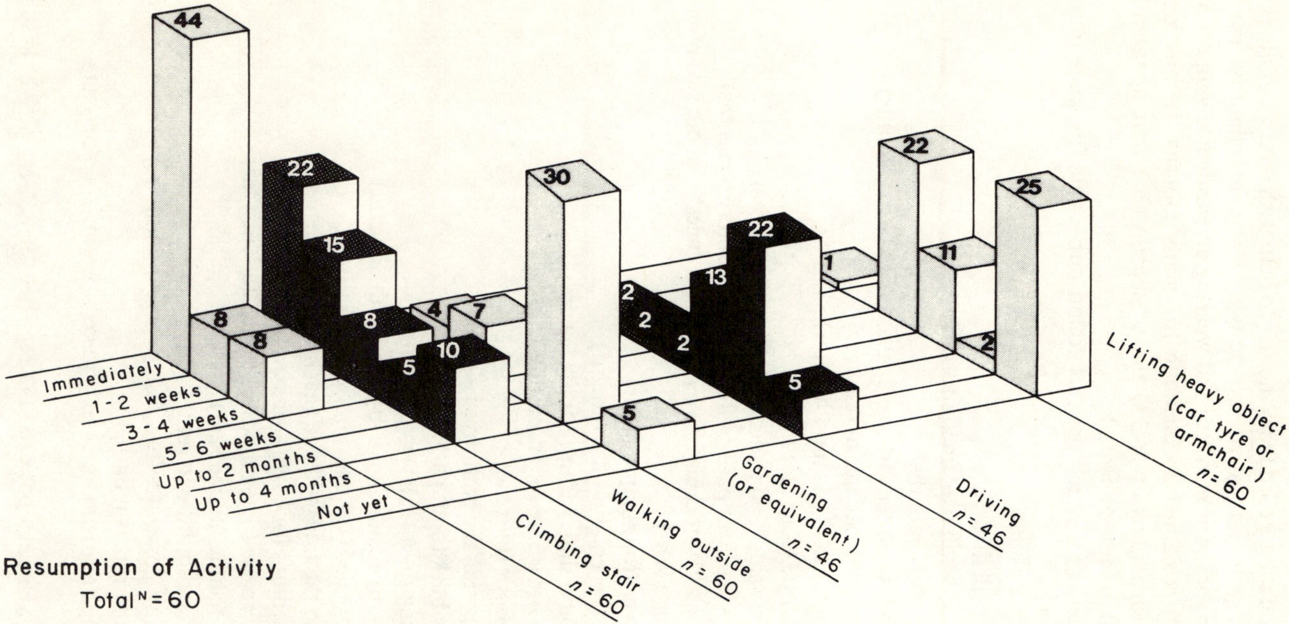
44
8
8
22
15
8
5
10
4
7
30
5
2
2
2
13
22
5
1
22
11
2
25
Immediately
1 - 2 weeks
3 - 4 weeks
5 - 6 weeks
Up to 2 months
Up to 4 months
Not yet
Climbing stair
n = 60
Walking outside
n = 60
Gardening
(or equivalent)
n = 46
Driving
n = 46
Lifting heavy object
(car tyre or
armchair)
n = 60
Resumption of Activity
Total N = 60

Figure 4

resorted to fixing a cord from the end to help with leverage. Others could only manage to get out of bed by lying flat and rolling on the floor. Pulling up socks for men (16) and wearing an elasticated support bra for women (4) remained problematic for many months. (Simple devices, available for pulling up socks, and a 'sleeping' bra were apparently not mentioned to these patients.)

Other activities which patients found impossible for some time after surgery were:

Sneeze (still dread it!)
Cough or laugh (still uncomfortable)
Lie flat (three months)
Put hands together with arms outstretched (two months)
Have sex (two patients at one year)
Work in the heat (six months later)
Concentrate (four months)
Lie on my side (two patients for 'some' months)
Sit up in bed (two patients for six weeks and two months)
Pull on elastic stockings (two patients for 'ages'—about two months)
Drive (at a year)
Bend over (for many months)
Bicycle (necessary—a postman!)
Dance and sing! ('Can't lift my leg up')
Wear a bra (three for six months)
Sweep floor (kills me)
Sit upright in the bath (lived alone)
Dry my back (one year later)
Polishing floor (still very difficult)
Raising my hands above my head (still difficult)
Make my bed (for one month)
Twist to the side (still at a year)
Paint ceilings (one year—decorator)
Have courage to go anywhere myself (at one year)
Go sea fishing (at one year)
Climb ladders (at one year)
Wear my corset for my disc problem (double problem to move around for six months)
Sleep upstairs (too much pain to get upstairs—at one year)

At one year, ten patients had regained their 'very active' leisure and social lives, 30 were moderately active, ten led their usual sedentary life (seven were in Group 1 and three were in Group 2) but a further 10 were frustrated by their inability to undertake their usual activities (six were in Group 3 and four in Group 2). For this last group, angina, sternal pain and leg swelling, numbness or pain were the reasons given for inactivity. Four of this group had seriously incapacitating and complicating conditions pre-operatively, the remainder did not have any such risk factors recorded.

Long-standing physical and psychological recovery

Two major physical problems were mentioned by patients—their leg after vein stripping and their sternotomy wound. Twenty patients had delayed leg wound healing and 14 still suffered from troublesome pain and swelling at one year post-operatively. Nineteen patients (13 of whom did not report any leg problem) complained of sternal pain, particularly during a twisting movement. This meant that two men gave up driving in this year and one other only resumed a few weeks before interview.

Twenty-one patients reported experiencing angina; for the majority this was only at times of extreme provocation such as heavy digging or watching an exciting film. Only four patients said this had not been improved by the operation.

Only seven patients reported high levels of anxiety and depression during this post-operative year. They all blamed physical ill-health, all were in Group 2 or Group 3, two were women and two were men who lived alone. When comparing emotion ratings across the three 'recovery' groups, the poor group (Group 3) were significantly more anxious (Kruskall Wallis analysis of variance $H = 13.2$, significant at the 0.001 level), although there were no such differences for depression ($H = 4.3$, NS). The women in particular felt more anxious and depressed in this post-operative year than pre-operatively.

Use of the self-concept scale was exploratory, but the 'helpless' dimension scores were significantly higher for Groups 2 and 3 than for those in the best recovery group (Kruskall Wallis $H = 9.9$, significant at the 0.001 level). No such differences were found for the 'positive' or 'negative' dimensions.

Return to work

At one year, 54 of these patients were in the working age group; 38 regained employment post-operatively—18 within three months and 20 at between 4 and 8 months (Figure 5). The reasons for unemployment

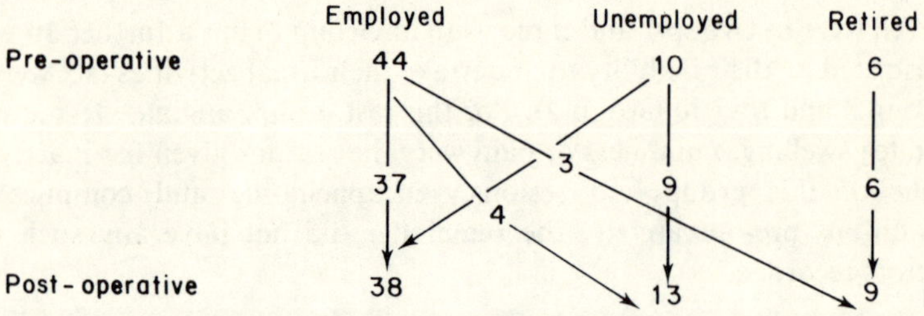

Figure 5 employment status. Total $N = 60$

post-operatively were usually a combination of 'not feeling well enough' and of being unable to find suitable work. Any work which involved a lot of standing, travelling or lifting seemed to mitigate against return to work. Of these 16, one was in his forties, 12 were in their fifties and three were in their early sixties and took early retirement. Their occupations are listed below under the three main factors (one clerk is omitted!) of the work that influenced their non-return.

Travelling	Standing	Physical
Pest-control officer	Shop assistant	Aircraft inspector
Travelling salesman	Teacher	Farmer
School officer	Gardener	Builder
Housing officer	Publican	Blasting foreman
Export manager	Hairdresser	Car mechanic

This list includes the six patients in the 'poor recovery' group and the remaining ten from the 'fair recovery' group. There were eight patients who had not returned to work who did not seem to suffer from definite physical symptoms. Half of them complained of fatigue and not being able to cope with a job. Their wives worked and they tended to do domestic jobs and help with looking after the family. Their mood scores tended to be greater (Mann–Whitney $z = 2.27$, significant at 0.01, for anxiety; $z = 1.01$, NS, for depression). The remainder were unable to find work and seemed genuinely distressed about this. They were characteristically unskilled and considered too 'risky' as future employees (This study was mainly done before the recession hit the employment market).

As was found in other studies, self-employed and unskilled people (12) suffered great financial hardship from illness and this encouraged an early return to work when possible.

Patient satisfaction

Forty-five patients said they got more enjoyment out of life since the operation. They did mention, however, that their wives were often protective and concerned that they were doing too much. Twenty-nine patients said they did not recall any advice about how much to do upon returning home and this made 14 of them rather anxious. General practitioners for ten of these patients dissuaded them from engaging in more active pursuits. Half the sample would have liked more opportunity to talk about their life at home and have specific guidance on activities.

Discussion

The majority of patients, all those in Groups 1 and 2, reported great benefits from this operation and all patients were very pleased to provide details of their post-operative recovery. The overall findings indicate that minor, non-cardiac problems seem to affect patients' progress. Only one previous report (Logue *et al.*, 1976) reviewed, discussed the problematic leg circulation, which prevented long periods of standing or walking often necessary for specific employment.

The poor rate of return to work is partly accounted for by the age of many patients—just before retirement. These patients certainly saw the operation as a watershed in their lives and, as they expected to be convalescent for several months, decided to give up work at the time of surgery; for instance, three women said they were encouraged by their husbands not to resume their jobs which had represented some social pleasure and economic freedom. Far from seeing the operation as giving them a new lease of life, it seemed to justify them taking things easy and their family taking on many of the heavy domestic chores, for a long time, if not permanently. Although these women were no older than the men in this sample, their recovery seemed much slower and they lacked 'courage' rather than the physical ability to resume some of their more active pursuits, like dancing.

There was genuine difficulty for four unskilled workers in regaining employment. When a medical examination was a necessary prerequisite they were not considered by employers. Success usually resulted in hiding their scar and working on temporary contracts. However, for eight others who said they had tried to find employment, it seemed that their motivation was not great and they also complained of fatigue and non-specific symptoms. Their work history was often unsatisfactory, with long periods of unemployment both before and during their treatment

Out-Patients' Questionnaire

(1) Was anyone at home to help you when you were discharged from hospital? ....

(2) What sort of help was necessary? ....
....

(3) What has been the most problematic aspect of your recovery at home? ....
....
....

(4) Did anyone either (a) encourage or (b) discourage your return to previous levels of activity? Who? (a) .... , ...
(b) .... , ...

(5) What were the most difficult activities for you to perform during your recovery, and why? ....
....
....

(6) (If applicable) Who made the decision that you should or should not go back to work? ....

(7) Is there anything you find particularly difficult about returning to work? ....
....
....

(8) Does your work involve long periods of standing, carrying weights or travelling?
Standing ....
Carrying weights ....
Travelling..................................

(9) Do any activities at home or work cause pain or breathlessness?..........
....

(10) What percentage would you give your present level of health (compared to someone of your own age)? Please ring an appropriate number

0 10 20 30 40 50 60 70 80 90 100%

(11) Now that some time has passed since you first became ill, do you feel that life has returned to normal? ....

(12) Is there anything else about your recovery you would like to mention?......
....
....

Figure 6

for angina. Their unemployment status was said to be distressing for them, although three of them seemed quite occupied with domestic and social activities. Others (Westaby *et al.*, 1979; Wallwork, 1978) have noted the relationship of pre- and post-operative unemployment patterns in this group of patients.

Patients' reports on lack of guidance for activity graduation at home cannot be taken at face value as they may well have forgotten such conversations. However, just under a quarter of this sample discussed this as an important omission, which created concern for them and their families. In the light of the numerous minor complications and a certain protectiveness by families, perhaps there should be more attention to pre-discharge counselling. Patients who were told 'walking is a good exercise' and 'to do a little more each day' found this useful. Certainly the spouse should be included when such advice is given!

Expectations that this operation should facilitate a pain-free, active existence should perhaps also be more publicized. Ten GPs were said to have prohibited more active pastimes or to have delayed return to work when patients requested this. This indicates undue caution which may be unjustified.

A systematic follow-up interview as employed in this study revealed many interesting insights into patients' difficulties upon returning home. Many of these could be prevented by some anticipation of these patients' needs. Patients could also provide answers to general questions reflecting their level of recovery, by completing a short questionnaire during the early follow-up visits to the out-patients' department. (This may follow the example provided in Figure 6.) Nurses in particular should learn more about patients' experiences at home and about their views of the operation in order to provide positive encouragement for activities and simple aids such as elastic leg supports or soft bras. Recovery for this group of patients was good on all the objective cardiological criteria when compared with other studies; it could perhaps be even better with more attention to certain practical, social and psychological aspects.

Acknowledgements

Much appreciation goes to the patients who helped with this study, to Dr. Redwood and Mr. Parker for their encouragement and to Sister Smith in the out-patients' department at St. George's Hospital.

References

Barnes, G. K., Oberman, A., Kouchoukos, N. T., and Ray, M. J. (1975). Changes in work status of patients undergoing saphenous vein by-pass surgery (SVBS). *Circulation,* **51, 52,** (Supplement II), 118.

Editorial (1979). Angina: The treatment revolution. *Lancet,* **ii**, 1167–1168.

European Coronary Surgery Study Group (1980). Prospective randomised study of coronary artery by-pass surgery in stable angina factors. *Lancet,* **i**, 491–495.

Gundle, M. J., Reeves, B. R., Tate, S., Raft, D., and McLaurin, L. P. (1980). Psychosocial outcome after coronary artery surgery. *American Journal of Psychiatry,* **137,** 1591-1594.

Lawrie, G. M., Morris, G. C., Howell, J. F., O'Gurra, J. W., Spencer, W. H., Cashion, W. P., Winters, W. L., Beazle, H. L., Chapman, D., Patterson, P. K., and Lic, J. P. (1978). Results of coronary by-pass more than 5 years after operation in 434 patients. *American Journal of Cardiology,* **40**, 665-672.

Logue, R. B., King, S. B., and Douglas, J. S. (1976). A practical approach to coronary artery disease, with special reference to coronary by-pass surgery. *Current Problems in Cardiology,* **1**, 1-53.

McIntosh, H. D., and Garcia, J. A. (1978). The first decade of aorta coronary by-pass grafting 1967-77. A review. *Circulation,* **47**, 3, 405-431.

Mendola, W. F., and Pelligrini, R. V. (1979). Quality of life and coronary artery by-pass surgery patients. *Social Science and Medicine,* **13A**, 457-461.

Mundth, E. D., and Austen, W. G. (1975). Surgical measures for coronary heart disease. *New England Journal of Medicine,* **293**, 13-20.

Oberman, A., and Kouchoukos, N. T. (1979). Working status of patients following coronary by-pass surgery. *American Heart Journal,* **98**, 132-133.

Pilowsky, I., Spence, N. D., and Waddy, J. L. (1979). Illness behaviours and coronary artery by-pass surgery. *Journal of Psychosomatic Research,* **23**, 39-44.

Porritt, D. (1979). *The Stress of Illness—Research Instruments.* Internal report. School of Community Medicine, University of New South Wales.

Preston, T. A. (1977). *Coronary Artery Surgery: A Critical Review.* Raven Press, New York.

Rimm, A. A., Barboriak, T. T., Anderson, A. J., and Simon, J. S. (1976). Changes in occupation after aorta coronary vein by-pass operation. *Journal of the American Medical Association,* **236**, 361-364.

Ross, J. K., Monro, J. L., Diwell, A. E., Mackean, J. M., Marsh, J., and Baker, D. J. P. (1981). The quality of life after cardiac surgery. *British Medical Journal,* **i**, 451-453.

Wallwork, J., Potter, B., and Cowes, P. K. (1978). Return to work after surgery for angina. *British Medical Journal,* **ii**, 1680-1681.

Westaby, S., Sapsford, R., and Bentall, H. N. (1979). Return to work and quality of life after surgery for coronary artery disease. *British Medical Journal,* **ii**, 1028-1031.

Willner, A. E., and Rabiner, C. J. (1979). Psychopathology and cognitive dysfunction five years after open heart surgery. *Comprehensive Psychiatry,* **20**, 409-418.

Wilson-Barnett, J. (1977). Patients' emotional reactions to hospitalisation. *Ph.D. Thesis.* University of London.

CHAPTER 6

Recovery from Stroke

LYNN BATEHUP

As with those suffering from ischaemic heart disease, patients with cerebrovascular problems form a very large group of chronically sick and potentially disabled people. Unlike the stress of recovery from surgery previously discussed, a stroke is a completely unexpected catastrophe. This may well account in part for the severe psychological problems which frequently occur and also for the unsatisfactory level of movement and activity which patients subsequently achieve. There are a host of considerations for planning care in both the early and later stages of recovery. Guidelines for practice to avoid permanent damage to limbs exist, although many of them have not been systematically assessed.

Much of this chapter gives details for continuous care of these patients rather than documenting evidence on poor levels of functional ability and social readjustment. This is an intentional contrast to the previous sections because it may well be the lack of guidance for staff on acute wards which leads to unnecessary morbidity. Stroke patients may stay on general medical wards for four to six weeks and receive only rudimentary exercises, partly as a result of mistaken beliefs that physiotherapists and speech therapists are the main agents of rehabilitation, but also because of the climate of acute care where other patients claim priority for nursing time. Opportunities to prevent the classic post-stroke posture of foot drop, leg drag and a contracted arm can be taken not only by those in specialized rehabilitation units. A combination of continuous and correct interventions explained here may do much to forestall long-term complications and hasten optimal recovery.

The word 'stroke' is in common usage throughout the world, but its exact meaning is poorly understood. The World Health Organization (1971) defines stroke as 'an acute disturbance of vascular origin causing disability lasting more than or death within 24 hours'. This definition does not make any differentiation between various causes of stroke, for which the medical and nursing treatments can differ considerably. In England and Wales in 1973, 80 583 people were certified as having died of cerebrovascular disease (Registrar General, 1975).

The prognosis following stroke is strongly influenced by the type of pathological lesion responsible. The two major causes of stroke are haemorrhage into brain tissue, and occlusion of cerebral or pre-cerebral arteries by thrombosis or embolus; subarachnoid haemorrhage, in comparison, causes few deaths. Very high mortality rates ranging from 60 to 90% have been observed in cases of intracerebral haemorrhage (Acheson and Fairbairn, 1970). The rates for cerebral infarction are lower at between 40 and 50%. During a three-year follow-up of stroke patients in the Manchester stroke study, Brocklehurst *et al.* (1978) found that only 37% of the patients survived to three years. A long-term study in America found that more than one half of the stroke victims died over the three-year period (Gresham *et al.*, 1979).

It is estimated that just over two in 1000 of the population has a stroke (Royal College of Physicians, 1974), rising to 20 per 1000 of the population in the age group 75–84 years. Thus, in a health district of 250 000 people there will be approximately 500 new stroke patients each year, the survivors joining the existing pool of handicapped people in the community.

The Effects of a Stroke

No two hemiplegic patients are quite alike, and if nursing care and medical management are to be effective they must conform to individual needs. These needs must be based on a thorough assessment of the patient's condition, which may consist of a motor paralysis with impaired postural control, sensory deficit, and some degree of intellectual deterioration.

The effects of stroke have been conveniently divided into motor and sensory deficits (Adams, 1971) and those important mental barriers to recovery described by Hurwitz and Adams (1972), which include speech difficulties, dementia, memory disturbances, motivation and true depression.

The close integration of motor and sensory components in functional movement makes it difficult to separate their effects, but in general motor defects include muscle weakness or paralysis, abnormalities in degree of muscle tone, and posture and balance disturbances.

Sensory, perceptual, and proprioceptive deficits include loss of sensation, visuospatial disturbances, defects of vision and hearing, and disorders of body image.

Speech impairment or communication disorders may be due to:

(1) Dysphasia: this covers all aspects of language and may include disorders in comprehension of spoken language, verbal expression, reading, writing, spelling, numbers, and telling the time (Meikle, 1981). Cryan Louis & Povse (1980) divide dysphasia into motor, or expressive dysphasia which affects the motor output of speech, and receptive or sensory dysphasia, which affects auditory comprehension and feedback of speech. Also included is global dysphasia which is a combination of these two types.
(2) Dysarthria is a disorder of muscle power of the tongue, lips and soft palate, which impairs movement of these organs; as a result intelligibility of speech, chewing and swallowing may be affected (Meikle, 1981).
(3) Dyspraxia is where there is a lack of voluntary control over the muscles of articulation or gesture.

Assessment of the Stroke Patient

Recovery from stroke may be regarded as occurring in three stages. The acute stage is seen as being up to the first two to three weeks following the completed stroke. The intermediate stage is most concerned with active rehabilitation, and can last as long as 18 months to two years. The third stage is the time required for social adaptation discussed in the next chapter. This entails return to social activities outside of the home, return to employment, and resumption of sexual activities.

The acute stage has the highest mortality rate, which may be in the region of 50%. Marquardsen (1976) states that type, size, and site of the cerebral lesion primarily decide the outcome of life, and irrespective of whether the lesion is haemorrhagic or thrombotic, it is the extent of damage to the vital centres in the brain stem that determines questions of life or death. Marquardsen found that the level of consciousness was a reliable prognostic sign, with those patients deeply unconscious on admission rarely recovering, and 80% with impaired consciousness dying.

It has been found that the risk of deep-vein thrombosis is much increased during the first 14 days after the stroke, with peak incidence on the fifth day, tailing off after 14 days (McCarthy, 1979), indicating that a hypercoagulable state exists for at least 14 days post-stroke. This necessitates a need to take notice of swelling and pain in a paralysed limb, and not to put it down simply to a belief that it is caused by loss of muscle tone or vascular tone.

In the elderly patient in the acute stage of stroke, death is not always caused by the cerebral lesion itself, but by other factors such as pneumonia, heart failure, or pulmonary embolism.

It is important to begin active rehabilitation as soon as possible, and this will follow stabilization of the patient's clinical condition. Rehabilitation should start with an assessment of motor and sensory function, orientation, communication, hearing and vision. This is also the time to assess the ability of the family or chief care giver to take part in the rehabilitation process.

Motor deficits

These are usually easily recognized. Problems can include: (1) Disturbance of postural, balance, and righting mechanisms. There is reduced ability to appreciate the body's position in space, to correct malalignment, and to place and hold the affected limbs. (2) Weakness or paralysis of muscles (loss of voluntary movement) on the side of the body contralateral to the cerebral lesion. (3) Variations in muscle tone. Immediately following the stroke the affected limbs are usually described as flaccid with sluggish or no reflex activity. There is then a gradual or sudden increase in tone and reflexes are brisk. The limbs are then described as spastic. The extent of spasticity varies from patient to patient.

In a study of hemiplegic patients Twitchell (1951) found that tendon reflexes became more active within 48 hours in some patients but in others this did not occur until between three and 29 days after the onset of hemiplegia, and gradually increased in intensity. It is also evident that spasticity is more pronounced in certain muscle groups, and that these are the muscle groups that oppose gravity. In the upper limbs spasticity is more pronounced in the scapular retractors and depressors, shoulder internal rotators and adductors, elbow flexors, forearm pronators, and wrist and finger flexors. This results in pulling down and backwards of the shoulder, flexion of the elbow, wrist and fingers, and the whole arm internally rotated. In the lower limbs spasticity tends to develop in the adductors and internal rotators of the hip, extensors of the knee and ankle plantar flexors and invertors. This produces a pulling upwards and backwards of the hip, an extended knee, the foot plantar flexed and internally rotated. The trunk and neck are also affected. The lateral flexors of the neck become spastic, drawing the head down to the affected shoulder, the trunk side flexors shorten the trunk of the affected side. This pattern of spasticity is common, and unless opposed will cause permanent joint abnormalities and loss of function.

Sensorimotor deficits

There is an increasing awareness that sensory and perceptual damage can be of greater significance for recovery than motor deficit alone, and this is reflected by the site of the lesion. Marquardsen (1976) found that patients with left-sided lesions made a better recovery than those with right-sided lesions.

The question of hemisphere function has long been under debate, and it is generally accepted that the left hemisphere is dominant for language function, and the right hemisphere greatly involved with functions of spatial orientation, perception of complex patterns, and the ability to construct complex configurations (Goldstein, 1974).

It is important that where there is speech difficulty an assessment of language function should be undertaken by a speech therapist. On the other hand, staff should be aware of the problems that may arise, so that communication between themselves and the patient can be maximized.

The process of assessment should include: the ability to comprehend spoken language; the ability to comprehend written language; the ability to use spoken language; the ability to name objects; the ability to repeat spoken language; the ability to write (Cryan and Povse, 1980).

Lesions of the right hemisphere are more often characterized by visuospatial difficulties, and by unilateral spatial neglect. Brain (1941) described the inattention for the left half of space in three patients with large right parietal lesions. This can be revealed in drawing and construction tests. For instance, some patients when asked to draw a clock face omit to draw the left side of the clock, or when drawing a house leave out the left side. Andrews *et al.* (1980), in a study which attempted to assess visuospatial and perceptual problems in hemiplegic patients through their drawing, found that the group with abnormal drawings had less muscular weakness, but that their activities in daily living functions were poorer than other stroke patients. This group, though, did continue to show recovery in these functions six months after the stroke. Disorders of body image are also more common in right-sided parietal lesions.

Depression

Storey (1976) in a study of 269 patients following subarachnoidal haemorrhage found that one quarter of these patients suffered from depression at some time following the onset of the illness, and this rate would appear to be as high in other types of stroke. It is important that all those caring for stroke patients should be aware of the possibility of a true depressive state and not too accepting of the patient's distress as a natural reaction.

Signs of depression, such as lowering of spirits and vitality, flattened mood, no response to pleasant events, sleep disturbances, loss of appetite and weight, may appear at any time throughout the recovery period. It may be difficult to recognize these symptoms, or to interpret them as a response to the patient's great loss of independence, social and family position, but it is part of the skilled activity of all health professionals to observe the patient's behaviour and to communicate with the family and friends who know best the patient's moods and possible response to stress and anxiety.

Hurwitz and Adams (1972) describe four behavioural changes associated with stroke illness which may be confused with poor motivation and depression:

(1) Emotional lability—the facile switching from joy to sadness.
(2) General loss of confidence.
(3) The decision to give up the struggle to regain function—that no more can be achieved.
(4) A condition known as emotional incontinence, which is quite different from emotional lability. This is characterized by sudden outbursts of weeping unrelated to the underlying mood, and provoked by the slightest stimulus. It is thought that this symptom seldom responds to treatment, and it is necessary to help the patient and relatives understand why it happens.

It was estimated in 1971 (Harris *et al.*, 1971) that there were 130 000 stroke victims living at home, and this is probably an underestimate; 71% of these survivors had severe disability. It is never easy to assess disability in stroke patients—the variations of possible functional abnormality are so numerous—but it may be possible by repeated structured assessment to identify them early and minimize the adverse effects.

Therapeutic Exercise used in Stroke Rehabilitation

It is no longer sufficient for a stroke patient to begin his rehabilitation struggling down a ward supported on either side by a nurse. It is being increasingly recognized that this approach does not take into account the neurophysiological aspects of learned movement, or the possible adverse effects of reflex activity. It is proposed to look briefly at several methods of therapeutic exercise, which can be grouped together under the heading, 'methods of facilitation and inhibition of motor activity'.

Flanagan (1967), in a review of such methods, numbered six factors common to all:

(1) Sensation and motion are intimately related to normal functions of the nervous system. These methods use sensation (sensory input) to some degree to facilitate or inhibit movement; the 'stretch simulus' is used by all methods.
(2) Each approach bases its methods on firm neurophysiological theory, and recognizes the importance of normal human motor development, both in treating those who are brain damaged at birth and those who suffer damage as adults.
(3) All methods recognize that early motor behaviour is influenced by reflex activity and use these reflexes during treatment to facilitate or inhibit voluntary movement. An understanding of reflex activity and pathways is essential.
(4) All methods use concepts of motor learning, such as repetition of activity, frequency of stimulation and use of sensory cues to help the learning process.
(5) All methods view the patient as a total person rather than focus on the impaired limbs.
(6) All methods rely on a close personal interaction between the therapist and patient.

The method for treating spastic paralysis was developed by Bobath and Bobath (1950) for the treatment of congenital and acquired hemiplegia and diplegia. This involves the neurophysiological concept that the nervous system evolves through a hierarchy of functions which range from stereotyped responses at spinal cord and lower brain stem levels, to more variable and selective ones which are integrated at subcortical and cortical levels; integration takes place between and at all levels. The basis of the treatment refers to the 'shunting rule' of Magnus (1926) and is expressed by Bobath (1979) as follows 'The changing state of the body musculature during movement is constantly reflected in the distribution of excitatory and inhibitory processes within the central nervous system. The body musculature, that is the proprioceptive system, therefore determines the motor output, i.e. the responses emanating from the central nervous system.' Peripheral sensory input is therefore used by the therapist to influence motor output. It is also stressed that, due to the release of subcortical and cortical inhibitory influences following brain damage, there emerge abnormal postural patterns which are under the influence of tonic and spinal reflexes. The spasticity that follows cortical damage is reduced by the use of reflex-inhibiting patterns. This method requires a knowledge of the normal sequential development of human motor behaviour, and uses it to treat the hemiplegic adult who has to relearn normal patterns of movement and posture.

The method described by Brunstromm (1970) for treatment of the adult hemiplegic patient emphasizes the effects of associated reactions which appear in the hemiplegic patient. These are defined by Walshe (1923) as tonic reflexes which occur in muscles deprived of voluntary control, and which have some degree of hypertonus. These movements which occur in the paralysed limb should not be regarded as movements in the strict physiological sense, but rather as variations in muscle tone and attitude elicited by forceful contraction of muscles. Associated reactions may be seen if a hemiplegic patient is asked to squeeze an object with the sound hand; it will be noted that spasticity will increase in the affected limbs.

Also important is the effect of tonic neck and labyrinthine reflexes on the character of these reactions, and the extension, flexion and synergistic patterns which the limbs adopt. Synergy is described by Brunstromm (1970) as muscles acting together as a bound unit in stereotyped patterns. This method evaluates the patient's level of function within the synergistic pattern, and uses various techniques to establish voluntary control of these stereotyped patterns of movement. When voluntary control is established, treatment employs facilitation techniques to help the patient break out of these set patterns. This is a highly individualized treatment and requires skilled therapists to carry it out.

The method developed by Dr. Herman Kabat (1977) in North America is known as proprioceptive neuromuscular facilitation. This method is based on the hierarchy of reflex actions integrated at various levels—spinal cord, mid-brain, and cortex—and that normal motor behaviour is closely interwoven with postural reflex mechanisms. Techniques of facilitation for maximum voluntary motion in neuromuscular re-education include maximal resistance, proprioceptive and other reflexes, and rhythmic stabilization (Kabat, 1977). Again in this, as in other neurophysiological methods, trained therapists are essential. Not discussed here are two other methods developed by Fay (1954) and Rood (1954).

The techniques of treatment developed by Berta Bobath have perhaps gained more popularity in the United Kingdom, especially in recent years. It is therefore proposed to look a little more closely at them with physiotherapy, nursing care and rehabilitation of the stroke patient in mind.

It is agreed by most authors writing about stroke rehabilitation that nursing care, especially in the early acute stage, is of utmost importance (Bobath, 1979; Johnstone, 1977). Nursing staff should be aware of the principles underlying therapeutic exercise in order that care and handling of stroke patients should not differ from that of the physical therapist. Failure to do this results in fragmented care, and confusion for the patient.

Bobath (1979) sees the problems arising from damage to the upper motor neurone as a derangement of the normal postural reflex mechanism. There is deviation from three fundamental prerequisites for normal motor function:

(1) Spasticity or flaccidity instead of normal levels of postural tone.
(2) The interplay of different muscle groups, agonists, antagonists, and synergists to give fixation for mobility, referred to as reciprocal innervation, is replaced by co-contraction of muscles. This results in the fixing of the patient in stereotyped postural patterns, with little or no selectivity of movement.
(3) Disturbances of the normal coordination of righting and equilibrium reactions.

The problem of spasticity is seen as the major one in the care of the stroke patient. Reference has been made to this earlier, but it is worth repeating that the onset and distribution of spasticity varies in each patient, and that, according to Twitchell (1951), the onset follows the pattern from distal to proximal, i.e. fingers and ankle upwards to shoulder and hip, and that when voluntary movement returned it was in the reverse direction—flexion of the shoulder and hip. The aim of treatment is to work towards achieving the patient's maximum function on both sides of the body, not to allow the patient to become a one-sided person using his sound side to compensate for the affected side. Bobath calls this 'compensatory rehabilitation'. Little emphasis is given to exercises to strengthen muscles and to maintain joint ranges as this is not seen as a major problem. The problem is seen as abnormal movement patterns which need to be released and changed.

Positioning and Handling of the Early Stroke Patient

The early days following a completed stroke are usually characterized by a reduction in muscle tone in the affected side, with spasticity becoming apparent in the ensuing days (Twitchell, 1951). It has been mentioned previously (Marquardsen, 1976) that level of consciousness is a poor prognosticator for recovery, but positioning of the patient whether in bed or in a chair is important and may affect ultimate functional ability (Bobath, 1979; D'Alton, 1974). Bad handling or man-handling of the patient may result in: unwanted increase in tone in the affected limbs; damage and pain to a vulnerable shoulder—subluxation; unilateral movements by the patient—compensatory action; loss of confidence by both patient and relatives, and nursing staff; back injuries to nursing staff.

The aims of the staff during early rehabilitation should be:

(1) Prevention of undue spasticity in the affected limbs.
(2) Handling and moving the patient in a controlled and therapeutic manner.
(3) To be aware of possible sensory and perceptual difficulties and help to minimize their effects.
(4) Help the patient make the psychological adjustment to his disability.
(5) Involve the chief carer in the programme from making the patient over-dependent.

Prevention of undue increase of spasticity in the affected limbs

Spasticity is usually seen first in the fingers and wrist followed by elbow and shoulder, and in toes and ankle followed by knee and hip. This is not a definitive pattern but occurs in large numbers of patients. If left untreated the spasticity will develop into definite patterns of abnormal posture (Bobath, 1979). In the upper limbs there will be flexion of the elbow, wrist and fingers, with depression and retraction of the shoulder. Shoulder extension is caused by depression of the muscle latissimus dorsi which pulls the shoulder downwards and backwards in internal rotation (Johnstone, 1977). In the lower limbs the tendency is for a pattern of extension to occur, in ankle, knee and hip, with external rotation of the leg. In some patients who have had an extensive infarct, flaccidity may persist, and when spasticity does appear it may cause a flexor tendency in the lower limbs. This will prevent the patient using the leg for standing or walking.

It is stated by Bobath (1979) that spasticity can be reduced by using 'reflex-inhibiting patterns' of posture, and that whether the patient is lying or sitting, in bed or chair, the limbs should be positioned to decrease spasticity. In general, the pattern for the trunk and upper limbs is extension of the neck and spine, elevation of the shoulder, extension of the elbow, wrist and fingers, abduction of the thumb, and external rotation of the arm at the shoulder. In the leg, it is abduction with flexion and protraction of the hip, extension of the knee and dorsiflexion of the foot (see Figures 7–11).

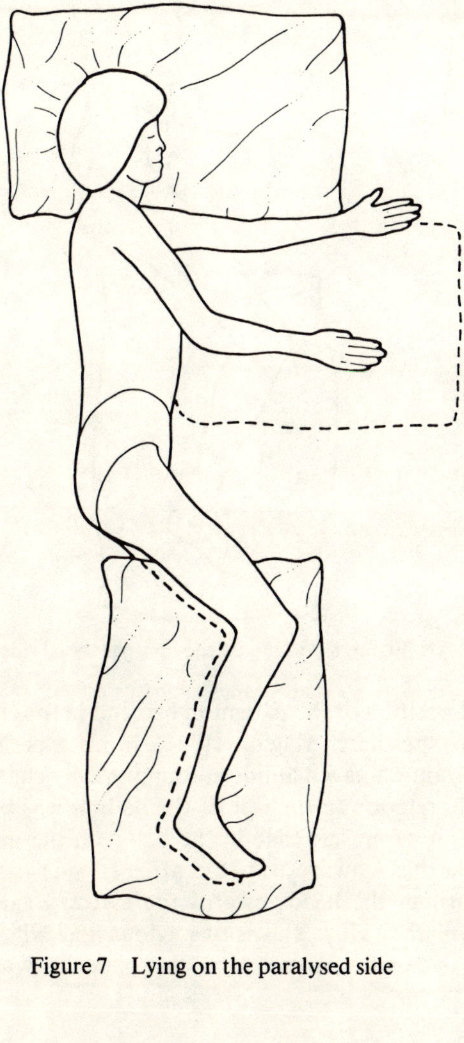

Figure 7 Lying on the paralysed side

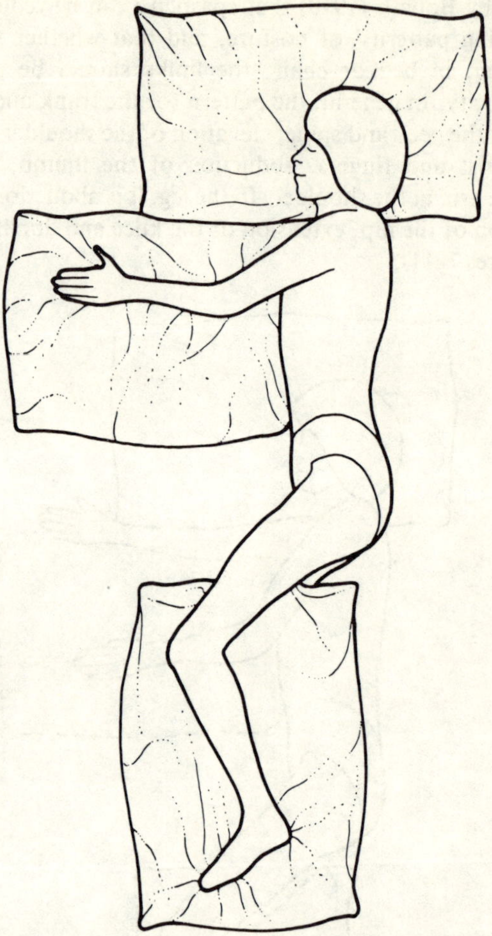

Figure 8 Lying on the non-paralysed side

The actual position of the patient in bed and in the chair is also crucial in minimizing spasticity. Magnus (1926), in his experiments on posture in prepared brain-damaged animals, found that by changing the position of the head in relation to the rest of the body it was possible to change the distribution of muscle tone in the body. In the hemiplegic patient, turning of the head away from the affected side increases the flexor spasticity, turning the head towards the affected side can reduce the spasticity (Bobath, 1979). This is of obvious note where patients ignore the affected side and always turn the opposite way. Lying on the

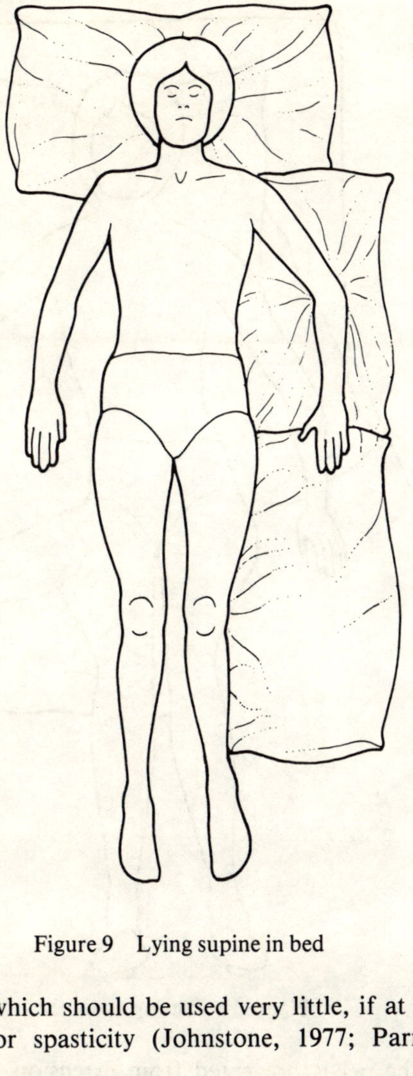

Figure 9 Lying supine in bed

back is a position which should be used very little, if at all, as it tends to increase extensor spasticity (Johnstone, 1977; Parry and Eales, 1976).

The positioning of stroke patients is very time-consuming as frequent adjustments have to be made. Two factors should be remembered. First, if the patient and his chief carers are involved and educated as to the importance of limb position, they can and are nearly always willing to participate in keeping the limbs correctly aligned. Secondly, the 'key points of control' are neck, spine, shoulder and pelvic girdles. Good alignment of head, neck and trunk with the arm kept externally

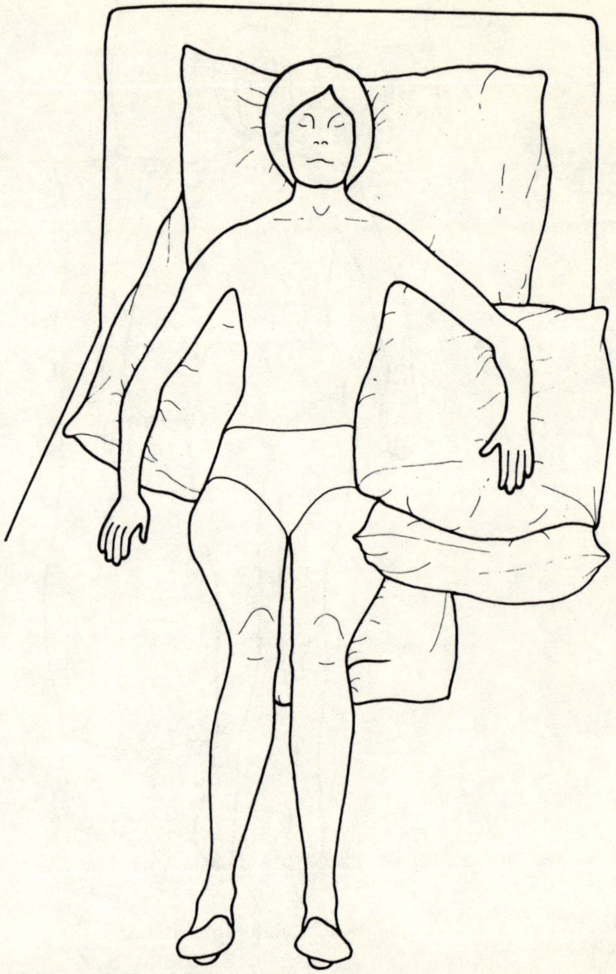

Figure 10 Sitting up in bed

rotated, and the pelvis prevented from extension, will go a long way towards preserving function.

Movement of the patient in a controlled and therapeutic manner

Movement of the patient will begin as soon as the clinical condition permits. Moving the patient should follow a sequential pattern. Just as a young child learns to roll, crawl, sit and stand in sequence, this should

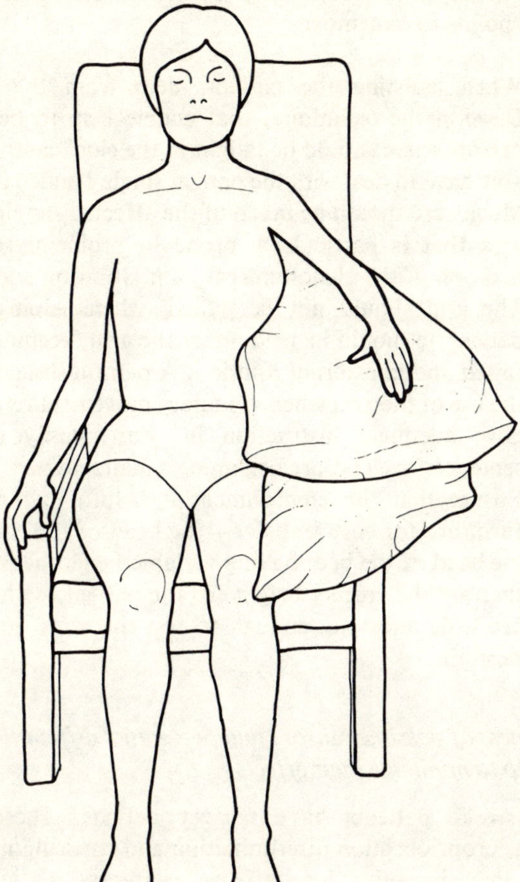

Figure 11 Sitting in a chair

also apply to the stroke patient as he has difficulty with balancing and righting mechanisms. It is bad practice to get a patient up out of bed without instructing him in rolling, sitting and propping himself up and balancing on the side of the bed. It is always a temptation to get the patient up and walking as quickly as possible with little consideration for the quality of movement, but in the long term this is unsatisfactory. It is beyond the scope of this chapter to go into detail about the techniques and programme of movement, but the reader is referred to two major texts (Bobath, 1979; Johnstone, 1977). However, listed below are some general points to remember:

(1) When assisting the patient, help from the affected side. Develop the techniques that enable help to be given by one person; these should be taught to the chief carer who will probably have to deal with the patient single-handed at home.
(2) Much care should be taken of the affected shoulder as this is an area that is particularly prone to problems, especially subluxation of the glenohumeral joint (Johnson and Olson, 1980). The arm should not be pulled; when helping to move the patient he should be held under the arm, keeping the arm itself raised and in external rotation. A painful shoulder can prevent the use of the arm when voluntary movement returns.
(3) Give adequate instruction in short, easily understandable sentences, well before beginning a manoeuvre.
(4) Ensure that the environment is helpful by: positioning the furniture for easy transfer—the head of the chair in line with the head of the bed; having variable-height beds; having chairs that are the correct height for the patient, with arm rests that are wide and long enough to rest the arms on in the correct position.

Awareness of possible sensory and perceptual difficulties and help to minimize their effects

Many stroke patients have sensory deficits. These include visual, hearing, proprioception discrimination and cortical integration (Adams, 1971). Proprioceptive loss affects awareness of joint position and movement. Disordered discriminative sensation interferes with touch localization and awareness of shape, size, form and texture (Adams, 1971). Impaired cortical integration affects the perception of the body image, resulting in unawareness, neglect, and denial of paralysis. It is necessary to differentiate between spatial neglect and visual-field defects. Andrews *et al.* (1980) found disorders of visuospatial function in 68 of 135 patients as revealed by disturbances of picture structure in drawings.

The first way that staff can help these patients is to be aware that these problems may exist and not to confuse them with poor motivation or 'not trying' (Marshall, 1971). The positioning of the patient and his furniture should be aimed at input to the affected side. Bed lockers should be placed on the affected side; this necessitates the patient reaching across to it, which produces rotation of the shoulders against the pelvis, an important reflex-inhibiting pattern called 'cross-facilitation' (Johnstone, 1977).

The special problems of unilateral spatial neglect and denial of disease are difficult to deal with. It is necessary to remind the patient frequently of the existence of the paralysed limbs. Where there is denial and delusionary descriptions of the limbs, Hurwitz and Adams (1972) advise that there should not be reinforcement and collusion by the carers.

Dysphasia is more common in left hemisphere lesions. Language function should be assessed by a speech therapist early on in the illness, as treatment should begin as soon as possible (Hopkins, 1975). If this is done the speech therapist will prove invaluable in helping the nursing staff and relatives understand the patient's handicap, and undertake specific speech and language rectification (Enderby, 1979). It has become more evident that, due to the small numbers of trained speech therapists, others would have to help with language retraining. Much valuable work has been done by speech therapists in setting up volunteer groups of non-professional people who go into the patient's home and help with speech therapy in a very fundamental way (Eaton Griffith and Miller, 1980). These types of groups are undoubtedly successful in supplementing the work of the speech therapist. Regular dyadic conversation for a set period each day has been shown to restore speech more rapidly than waiting for the patient to initiate this. It apparently requires nothing more sophisticated than interest and motivation from both individuals.

Helping the patient make the psychological adjustment to disability

A stroke renders to the once intact person a new and incomplete body image; in addition to this he may lose many practical and expressive functions, such as control of elimination and sexual function. This may be looked upon as a period of loss, combining grief, depression and anxiety (Ripeckyj and Lazarus, 1980).

Grief is a natural reaction to loss or bereavement, and may be described as the process of psychological adjustment needed to cope and eventually adapt to the loss.

Bereavement is defined by Carlson and Blackwell (1978) as 'the loss of a person, thing, body part, idea, model or relationship in which dependency plays a critical role.' Different stages in the grief reaction have been described by Kubler Ross (1969) as denial, anger, bargaining, depression and acceptance; and by Parkes (1972) as alarm, searching, mitigation, anger and guilt, and gaining new identity. These descriptions will not apply to all grieving persons or be as clear-cut as described; there will also be much overlap between the various stages. Carlson and Blackwell (1978) describe the stages through which grieving persons may go:

(1) Pre-crisis phase. For the stroke patient this may occur as a transient ischaemic attack, a warning of impending catastrophe. Care can be aimed towards helping the patient cope, and mobilizing resources to mitigate further episodes.
(2) Impact and shock phase. This follows the catastrophe and may prevent the person from perceiving the reality of the situation. This also applies to a spouse, a wife who has always relied on her husband to take care of everything. Euphoria and feelings of indifference are commonly reported at this stage. The carer needs to be aware of this, and help and guide the patient and family member.
(3) Retreat. Initial awareness of the significance of the loss may be intolerable to either the patient or relatives, and this may be where avoidance behaviour becomes evident. Denial is a commonly used defence mechanism, an adaptive manoeuvre used to reduce anxiety (Keining, 1978). This may be exhibited as intense activity, avoidance of discussion of anything related to the disability, or refusal of treatment as being unnecessary. Staff at this time should not push the patient into facing problems head on; observe for signs of acceptance and try not to reinforce the denial.
(4) Acknowledgement. This phase is characterized by confrontation with the realities of loss; this applies to both the patient and family members. This phase may be of longer duration than the others. Emotions of anger, depression, guilt and bitterness may be expressed. Guilt is often felt by a wife who makes a remark such as 'if only I hadn't pushed him so hard'. Anger by the patient may be focussed on those caring for him, or on the nearest relatives. Intervention for helping individuals cope with these mixed emotions is directed towards an understanding for the patient of the sadness and depression that is being felt. Time should be allocated for therapeutic listening.
(5) Acceptance and adaptation. As this stage implies, it is the time the individual comes to terms with his changed state. More energy is now being expended on behaviour to enable him to function to his best ability. Nursing care is now focussed on helping to set realistic goals for the future in order to obtain maximum return of function and social integration.

Every individual differs in the extent to which these emotions may be experienced, and in the brain-damaged person it is sometimes difficult to assess emotional problems because of possible interference with intellectual function. Nevertheless, stroke is a catastrophic event in a person's life, and a loss-reaction to it should be expected.

Involve the chief carer in the programme from the start

It has been the personal experience of the author that the inclusion of the person who is going to care for the stroke patient at home in the rehabilitation programme from the beginning is of great importance and has the advantages of:

(1) Helping relatives to cope with any possible guilt feelings they might have by their active participation in the recovery process.
(2) Helping the family to unite and direct their goals to the benefit of the patient.
(3) Learning techniques that enable the family to help confidently when discharge comes.
(4) If the family have confidence in their own ability and have some knowledge of the recovery process, they are less likely to over-protect the patient, and will encourage dependence.

Of course it will not be every patient who has a relative or friend who is able to help with rehabilitation, because of physical frailty, but this should not preclude them from involvement in the activities. Their presence at mealtimes, exercise sessions, transfer activities, dressing, and all the many other activities taking place is invaluable in giving them an insight into the problems faced by the patient, and ultimately themselves. There is a danger that, once home, the patient may be made over-dependent by a relative who is unaware of the function achieved in hospital. A study by Garraway *et al.* (1980), comparing functional ability in two groups of stroke patients—one group from a stroke unit and the other group from a medical unit—found on one-year follow-up that the higher percentage of independent patients discharged from the stroke unit as compared with the medical unit had been reversed. On reassessment, 57% of medical unit patients were independent, and 55% of stroke unit patients were independent. It seems that as follow-up progressed, independent stroke unit patients were allowed to do less and less, and dependent medical unit patients were allowed to do more. It was thought that factors contributing to these results were, first, the greater protection given to the stroke unit patients by their relatives in not allowing them to carry out activities of which they were capable. Despite the greater involvement of these relatives during hospital stay, the question arises as to adequate orientation and instruction given to them regarding future rehabilitation prospects following discharge and the need to maintain the abilities gained during the acute stage. This indicates a clear need for patient and family education not on an ad hoc basis, but as part of a carefully planned programme including a discharge care plan. The second contributory factor was the larger number of medical unit patients who were assessed as dependent at discharge but who consequently gained their independence during follow-up. This group spent less time in hospital than other medical unit patients, and it is thought they had not reached their full potential at discharge.

Hamrin (1981) reports on her study of 56 stroke patients who were randomly assigned to either an experimental group (E) or a control group (C). The aims of the study were to find out whether a systematic activation programme in the daily nursing care of stroke patients in medical wards, in conjunction with an educational programme on stroke for staff (experimental group), would result in: improvement of the functional capacity of the stroke patients one year after the stroke; improvement of the situation of stroke patients from a physical as well as a psychosocial point of view from the acute stage up to the end of three months after the stroke; improvement of the attitudes of staff concerning activation and understanding of stroke patients. Further aims were development of an activation programme in nursing, development and evaluation of instruments to measure functional capacity, and development of an educational programme for stroke activation.

The experimental group received individualized activation programmes mainly within the first four weeks. The following factors were amongst those emphasized: psychological activation, verbal communication, prophylaxis against contractures, movement therapy, ambulation, and activities of daily living. Staff on the experimental wards received a series of lectures given over a period of time concentrating on various aspects of stroke care. The control group received the usual care given to stroke patients on a general medical ward.

The results are interesting in that they resemble those of Garraway *et al.* (1980). Measurement of functional capacity using a 92-score Activity Index at three months showed that the two groups had progressed equally, and that the experimental group showed a tendency to benefit while the activation programme was being practised. At one-year follow-up, no long-term effects of the activation programme could be proved.

Again, this is a strong indication for much longer-term rehabilitation programmes including structured education for care givers in order that rehabilitation should continue following discharge, at home and in special centres. Much valuable work can be done by relatives and volunteers, coordinated by primary health workers.

It is suggested by Mulhall (1980) that relatives caring for the patient will usually require the following: factual information, practical suggestions about what to do and what not to do; the opportunity to crystallize ideas by talking about feelings and difficulties.

There is a growing interest in the rehabilitation of the stroke patient, especially among the physiotherapy, occupational therapy, and speech therapy professions. Nurses remain as the group who spend more time with the patients than any other, and are therefore in a position to play a major part in the recovery process. Evaluative research is necessary in this field of nursing intervention. There is a need to develop a nursing tool to measure the extent that hemiplegic limbs are being positioned to avoid increasing spasticity, so that some indication is given of how treatment in the acute stages effects eventual functional ability. Research could also be directed towards ways in which nursing intervention could help towards the psychological adjustment being experienced by patient and relatives. Only in this way can the nursing contribution to stroke recovery be placed on a more scientific footing.

References

Acheson, R. M., and Fairbairn, A. S. (1970). Burden of cerebrovascular disease in the Oxford area in 1963–1964. *British Medical Journal*, **ii**, 621.

Adams, G. F. (1971). Capacity after stroke. *British Medical Journal*, **i**, 91–93.

Andrews, K., Brocklehurst, J. C., Richards, B., and Laycock, P. J. (1980). The prognostic value of picture drawings by stroke patients. *Rheumatology and Rehabilitation*, **19**, 180–188.

Bobath, B. (1979). *Adult Hemiplegia: Evaluation and Treatment.* Heinemann Medical Books, London.

Bobath, K., and Bobath, B. (1950). Spastic paralysis: treatment of by the use of reflex inhibition. *British Journal of Physical Medicine*, **13**, 121–127.

Brain, R. (1941). Visual disorientation with special reference to lesions of the right hemisphere. *Brain*, **64**, 244–272.

Brocklehurst, J. C., Andrews, K., Morris, P. E., Richards, B., and Laycock, P. J. (1978). Medical, Social and Psychological Aspects of Stroke. Department of Geriatric Medicine, University of Manchester. Unpublished report.

Brunstromm, S. (1970). *Movement Therapy in Hemiplegia. A Neurophysiological Approach.* Harper & Row, New York.

Carlson, C. E., and Blackwell, B. (1978). *Behavioural Concepts and Nursing Intervention.* J. B. Lippincott, Philadelphia.

Cryan Louis, M., and Povse, S. M. (1980). Aphasia and endurance: Considerations in the assessment and care of the stroke patient. *Nursing Clinics of North America,* **15**, 265–282.

D'Alton, A. (1974). Physiotherapy in the early rehabilitation of the hemiplegic patient. *Nursing Mirror,* **139**, 62–66.

Eaton Griffith, V., and Miller, C. L. (1980) Volunteer stroke scheme for dysphasic patients with stroke. *British Medical Journal,* **281**, 1605–1607.

Enderby, P. (1979). How does speech therapy work? *Practitioner,* **223**, 796–799.

Fay, T. (1954). The use of pathological and unlocking reflexes in the rehabilitation of spastics. *American Journal of Physical Medicine,* **33**, 347–352.

Flanagan, E. M. (1967). Methods for facilitation and inhibition of motor activity. *American Journal of Physical Medicine,* **46**, 1006–1011.

Garraway, W. M., Aktar, A. J., Hockey, L., and Prescott, R. J. (1980). Management of acute stroke in the elderly: follow up of a controlled trial *British Medical Journal,* **281**, 827–829.

Goldstein, G. (1974). *The Use of Clinical Neuropsychological Methods in the Lateralization of Brain Lesions.* In S. Dimond and J. G. Beaumont (Editors), Hemisphere Function in the Human Brain. Elek Science, London.

Gresham, G. E., Phillips, T. F., Wolf, P. A. McNamara, P. M., Kannel, W. B., and Dawber, T. R. (1979). Epidemiologic Profile of long term stroke disability: The Framingham study. *Archives of Physical Medical Rehabilitation,* **60**, 487–491.

Hamrin, E. (1981). Activation of patients with stroke in clinical nursing care—effects on patients and staff. *Abstracts of Uppsala Dissertations in Medicine,* 407.

Harris, A. I., Cox, E., and Smith, C. R. W. (1971). *Handicapped and Impaired in Great Britain,* Part I. H.M.S.O., London.

Hopkins, A. (1975). The need for speech therapy for dysphasia following stroke. *Health Trends,* **7**, 58–60.

Hurwitz, L. J., and Adams, G. F. (1972). Rehabilitation of hemiplegia: Indices of assessment and prognosis. *British Medical Journal,* **i**, 94–98.

Johnson, K., and Olson, E. (1980). Application of the Bobath principles for nursing care of the hemiplegic patient. *Journal of the Association of Rehabilitation Nurses,* **31**, Mar./Arp., 8–11.

Johnstone, M. (1977). *The Stroke Patient: Principles of Rehabilitation.* Churchill-Livingstone, London and Edinburgh.

Kabat, H. (1977). Studies in Neuromuscular Dysfunction. In O. D. Payton, S. Hirt and R. A. Newton (Editors), *Neurophysiologic Approaches to Therapeutic Exercise.* F. A. Davis, Philadelphia.

Kiening, Sister M. Martha (1978). Denial of Illness. In C. Carlson and B. Blackwell (Editors), *Behavioural Concepts and Nursing Intervention.* J. B. Lippincott, Philadelphia.

Kubler Ross, E. (1969). *On Death and Dying.* Macmillan, New York.

Magnus, R. (1926). General static reactions of the midbrain animal. *Lancet,* **ii**, 585–588.

Marquardsen, J. (1976). Follow up of stroke patients. Age and ageing. *VII European Congress of Clincial Gerontology,* Manchester, 10–14 September, 1974.

Marshall, J. (1971). Neurological deficit after stroke. *Modern Geriatrics,* **1**, 6, 380–382.

McCarthy, S. T. (1979). Vascular complications of stroke. *Practitioner,* **223,** 675–677.

Meikle, M. (1981). Listen I want to tell you something. *Nursing Times,* August 5 Supplement, **7**:10–13, 14.

Mulhall, D. (1980). Counselling relatives towards a helping relationship. *Geriatric Medicine,* **10**, 4, 39–42.

Parkes, C. M. (1972). *Bereavement: Studies of Grief in Adult Life.* Basic Books, New York.

Parry, A., and Eales, C. (1976). Handling the early stroke patient at home and in the ward. *Nursing Times,* **72**, 1680–1683.

Ripeckyj, A., and Lazarus, L. W. (1980). Family guide to the problems of the stroke patient. *Geriatrics,* **35**:Oct, 47–48.

Rood, M. S. (1954). Neurophysiological reactions as a basis for physical therapy. *Physical Therapy Review,* **34**, 444–449.

Royal College of Physicians (1974). *Report of the Geriatric Working Group on Strokes.* London.

Storey, P. (1976). Depression after stroke. *Chest, Heart and Stroke Journal,* **1**, 14–17.

Twitchell, T. E. (1951). The restoration of motor function following hemiplegia in man. *Brain,* **74**, 443–480.

Walshe, F. M. R. (1923). On certain tonic or postural reflexes in hemiplegia with special reference to the so called associated movements. *Brain,* **46**, Part 1.

World Health Organization (1971). Cerebrovascular diseases: Prevention treatment and rehabilitation. *WHO Technical Report Series,* No. 469.

CHAPTER 7

Problems of Definition and Measurement in Longer-Term Recovery

CECILY J. PARTRIDGE

Recovery from illness implies a restoration to a state of health, and for many patients a return to health is the expected result. However, when irreversible damage to systems or structures of the body has been sustained as a result of disease or trauma, a full return to the pre-morbid state is not possible. Recovery for these patients consists of two overlapping phases—an initial period of natural recovery where some damaged tissues resume their function, followed by an adjustment of the individual to the irreversible changes that have occurred. This second phase may take place over a considerable length of time and will be influenced by a number of different factors—physical, social and psychological.

The number of people with conditions involving some residual defects is considerable. Harris (1971) estimated that there were over three million people aged sixteen or over living in the community who had some residual physical, mental or sensory impairment. In their terms impairment was 'lacking a part or all of a limb or having a defective limb, organ or mechanism of the body'. A substantial proportion of patients in this group have limited physical functioning as a result of their condition: for example, those suffering from the effects of trauma, heart disease, arthritis or stroke. Some of these conditions are expected to progress and therefore there is a continuing process of adaptation to the changes that are occurring.

There have been a number of problems in investigating and assessing patients with this type of physical disability and perhaps the lack of an appropriate framework for considering the consequences of long-term and chronic disease is the most fundamental. The medical model of disease, with the emphasis on identifying pathological processes, deciding on a diagnosis and instituting appropriate treatment, is not suitable for conditions where prevention or cure is not possible.

Another major problem that has impeded progress in this area is the lack of general agreement on the use of terms to describe the results of disease or trauma for the patients with residual physical disability. Sainsbury (1973) discusses motor capacity, self- and household care, physical dependence and the capacity for work, all under the heading of disability, while Jefferys *et al.* (1969) describe motor capacity and physical dependence as impairment, and use the terms impairment and limitation synonymously. Stichbury (1975) investigates the assessment of locomotor ability under the heading of 'disability' following head injury, and Katz *et al.* (1970) consider any restriction of function of any activity of daily living as being part of the dynamics of disability. Harris (1971) uses only the terms handicap and impairment.

Recognizing the confusion in this area, which was both conceptual and semantic, the World Health Organization (1980) proposed an International Classification of Impairments, Disabilities and Handicaps (ICIDH). This new classification introduced both concepts and definitions of impairment, disability and handicap, and provided a framework for understanding the consequences of disease, particularly for chronic, progressive or irreversible disorders. It is supplementary to the International Classification of Diseases (ICD) (World Health Organization, 1969), which is a practical scheme of classification of disease and injury for general statistical use.

The three codes proposed in the ICIDH are defined as follows: impairment is concerned with abnormalities of body structure and of the function of organs and systems; disability reflects the consequences of impairment in terms of performance and activity by the individual; and handicap is concerned with the disadvantages experienced by the individual as a result of impairment and disabilities. Impairment resembles the disease terms used in the ICD code, and is considered as a threshold phenomenon, judged to be either present or absent; no measurement of impairment is suggested, though the assessment and measurement of both disability and handicap are discussed. If this new classification is generally accepted it should provide a framework for examining the consequences of disease for patients with long-term, chronic and progressive diseases.

Measurement of the consequences of disease is complex and there are, at present, few generally acceptable and reliable tools available. Most measurements of limitation of activity or function, whether described as impairment, disability, or handicap, have been developed for one of two purposes—either for population statistics (Jefferys *et al.*, 1969; Harris, 1971; Sainsbury, 1973), or to assess an individual's level of function at specific times (Katz *et al.*, 1970; Stichbury, 1975; Whiting and Lincoln, 1980).

Those that have been developed to obtain information from the total population about levels of physical ability are not suitable for monitoring progress in the recovery of physical skills, because they lack the necessary sensitivity and include many items inappropriate for patients in hospital during the early stages of recovery; for example, cooking, shopping, going on holiday (Harris), preparing and cooking a hot meal, running to catch a bus, hanging out the washing (Sainsbury). Jefferys *et al.* (1969) used activities which simulated daily living activities; for example, 'grasp a weighted tumbler using thumb and two fingers, raise to mouth level'.

Scores indicate whether or not the patient performs the activity in the stated manner, but make no allowance for gradations in performance; nor do such scales take into account the actual defects or dysfunction of body structure or systems. The scales used by Stichbury involved a series of movements which followed a developmental sequence, starting with the patient being tested lying down and progressing through sitting to standing. These assessments were specifically developed to record progress in patients with a neurological condition. Few of these tests give evidence of the reliability of their methods of assessment and measurement when used with patients, and therefore it is difficult to interpret the results of studies where they have been used.

More recently developed tools of measurement do provide evidence of objectivity. Sheikh *et al.* (1979)—Activities of Daily Living Index—and Lincoln and Leadbitter (1979)—Assessment of Motor Function—both provide evidence of the reliability of their tests when used with a specified population of stroke patients. Lincoln's is one of the very few tests able to demonstrate the unidimensional and cumulative nature of the scale, and a total score in this case does have some meaning.

Although scoring an individual's performance on a scale can provide a method of monitoring change, it is important to consider exactly what is being measured. Many early tests made the assumption that the tests were measuring the patient's actual ability. However, any test of performance can only measure what the individual does do in response to a request on that occasion. Many different factors may influence performance; such things as mood, the desire to cooperate with the tester, or the time of day or previous activities may all alter results. It is important to remember that there may be different levels of disability associated with any given impairment, and how the individual performs will represent both the actual physical limitations imposed by his condition and the way in which he perceives and reacts to these changes.

There have been few investigations which have attempted to study factors which affect this longer-term recovery and account for the commonly observed differences which occur in the rate and type of recovery achieved by patients with conditions of similar severity. Approaches to treatment and management tend to relate to the patient's diagnosis and to the clinical signs, but for patients with disorders which involve coping with physical incapacity it may be important to examine the patient's reactions to his condition as well as to the condition itself.

Lazarus (1974) stressed the link between the way an individual appraises a stressful situation and his ability to cope with that situation. The onset of a condition such as a stroke must be regarded as intrinsically stressful but may be perceived and appraised in different ways. In preliminary work by Partridge (1982), working with patients who had suffered a stroke of at least moderate severity, wide variations in both primary and secondary appraisal were demonstrated. When paralysis first occurred, some patients viewed it immediately as something serious; others felt that it was possibly transitory and therefore not serious. On secondary appraisal, when there had been time to consider the implications of their condition, there was still great variation. Asked to rate the seriousness of their condition, some patients said they were not ill at all and were, in fact, perfectly healthy but their condition was a nuisance. Others, however, saw themselves as very ill and found it difficult to find words to express the awfulness of what had happened to them, one patient stating that she thought it was the most terrible thing that could happen to anyone. Where adaptation to change is involved as it is in coping with physical disability, it might be expected that the individual's perceptions would influence the type and extent of coping behaviour. Early results suggest that this is the case, and that patients who saw their condition as less severe were more likely to cope more effectively and regain independent performance of activities sooner than those who perceived their condition in more extreme terms.

Because impairment is considered as a threshold phenomenon and not subject to measurement, the assessment of the severity of stroke in any patient must relate to measurements of disability and handicap. There may be variations in any one patient's performance and it must be remembered that results will only reflect what he does on the occasion of the test—it cannot be presumed that performance on any one occasion reflects the individual's actual physical ability. Another question which warrants consideration is whether performance in a test situation reflects the level of performance that can be achieved in a real-life situation, which is, of course, often the primary purpose of the test. Sheikh *et al.* (1979) found a considerable discrepancy between performance in a test situation and the patients' estimates of their own activities at home, the activities at home falling well below those indicated by the results of tests in hospital.

If patients with different kinds of disabilities and handicaps are to be helped to function at a level which is optimum for them, it is essential that tools of measurement are developed which are reliable and sensitive enough to reflect change when it occurs. Careful monitoring of longer-term recovery is required to obtain a more complete picture of changes that occur over a longer time period. Only by doing this can the effectiveness of any intervention be adequately assessed.

References

Harris, A. I. (1971). *Handicapped and Impaired in Great Britain.* H.M.S.O., London.

Jefferys, H., Millard, J. B., Hyman, M., and Warren, M. D. (1969). Tests for measuring motor impairment in prevalence studies. *Journal of Chronic Diseases,* **22**, 303–319.

Katz, S., Ford, A. B., Moskowitz, R. W., Jackson, B. A., and Jaffe, M. W. (1970) An Index of Activities of Daily Living. *Gerontologist,* **10**, 20–30.

Lazarus, R. S. (1974). Psychological stress and coping in adaptation and illness. *International Journal of Psychiatry in Medicine,* **5**, 321–333.

Lincoln, N., and Leadbitter, D. (1979). Assessment of motor function in stroke patients. *Physiotherapy,* **65**, 48–51.

Partridge, C. J. (1982). A study of cognitive and emotional factors as predictors of recovery. Manuscript in preparation.

Sainsbury, S. (1973). Measuring disability. *Occasional Papers on Social Administration,* No. 53. Bell, London.

Sheikh, K., Smith, D. S., Meade, T. W., Goldenberg, E., Brennan, P. J., and Kinsella, G. (1979). Repeatability and validity of modified Activities of Daily Living Index in studies of chronic disability. *International Rehabilitation Medicine,* **1**, 51–58.

Stichbury, J. (1975). Assessment of disability following severe head injury. *Physiotherapy,* **61**, 268–272.

Whiting, S., and Lincoln, N. (1980). An ADL assessment for stroke patients. *Occupational Therapy,* **43**, 44–46.

World Health Organization (1969). *International Classification of Diseases (revised).* Geneva.

World Health Organization (1980). *International Classification of Impairments, Disabilities and Handicaps.* Geneva.

CHAPTER 8

Future Research and Practical Implications

From reviewing this work there seems to be a glaring need for further knowledge to make recommendations for helping recovery and for facilitating both management and continuity in the longer-term, post-hospital phase. Although we have chosen specific areas to illustrate the inadequacy of both knowledge and care, readers may consider that other areas are equally worthy of attention. The subject of recovery is wide-ranging and complex and relies on both patients' and health service resources. Many health workers have an influence on recovery and the professions tend to specialize in certain aspects, so that overall co-ordination is sometimes lacking. A comprehensive understanding of the effect of, and recovery from, illness on the individual necessitates multidisciplinary research combining physical and behavioural sciences, and multiprofessional research teams. Although this type of research is most likely to provide a sound basis for the preparation, treatment, care and after-care of patients, it is also the most expensive research in time and money and the most difficult to set up, as it involves crossing boundaries between different disciplines and different environments. However, even without further research there is scope for the practices of specialized centres of excellence to be applied more widely. In this book we have tried to suggest some positive contributions, several of which refer to more than one group of patients.

When attempting to propose remedies or initiatives, these should be based on sound research. For many aspects there are as yet only indications from research and therefore both physiological and psychosocial studies are needed. Some research-based guidelines on advice are in existence; for example, 'Medical Aspects of Fitness to Drive' produced by the Medical Commission on Accident Prevention (Raffle, 1976). Other research has attempted to understand the factors which influence the length of stay in hospital (Griffiths *et al.*, 1979; Simpson *et al.*, 1977) and return to work (Strasser, 1977; Bourke *et al.*, 1981). Having said this, one cannot ignore the individual variations in recovering from the same problems, and identifying those at risk of poorer psychological responses in the longer term is not really systematically possible without more prospective studies and more refined and valid measures of recovery.

Recommendations for Future Recovery Care

Two important areas—patient teaching and continuity of care—should be considered to have fundamental influences on patient recovery. Both are inadequate at present and both require staff effort, time and an awareness of patients' needs. Several research studies already reviewed show that more teaching and continuity of care is beneficial.

Preparation for discharge from hospital

It should be recognized that, with an increasingly rapid turnover on surgical wards, in particular, many patients are discharged at an earlier stage of the recovery process than before. Their needs for preparation at this time are therefore greater. Preparation involves anticipating those needs, giving information and instruction and coordinating arrangements for continued care.

Patient teaching should start a few days before discharge and should also involve the spouse or nearest relative (Roberts, 1975). Most of all, it should give the patient an accurate picture of the staff's expectation for their optimum state of health. It should also provide a realistic picture of the most likely experiences the patient will have on return home and during recovery. The principle was discussed in Chapter 3. Where anticipation accords to the experience this reduces anxiety and gives the patient an increased feeling of control. Any routine symptoms which may occur will be understood and not be accompanied by irrational fears and unnecessary invalidism.

Principles of patient teaching have been carefully outlined by Redman (1975). The patient should be motivated to learn, feel relaxed with the 'teacher', and should not be overloaded with information. Redman suggests planning to discuss no more than three major issues at any one time, to follow stages agreed by the patient, and to make a written copy of the information for the patient and his family for use in the future. Each session should begin by answering questions and by reiterating the goals of that session and the content of those previously conducted.

Table 6 Teaching plan after major surgery, prior to discharge

CONTENT	GOAL
(1) *Three days prior to discharge, five days after surgery*	
(with Nurse M and Mr. and Mrs. P)	
i. Introduction to teaching for return home—goal setting and plan. Ask for any questions of current concern.	
ii. Clarify any aspects of surgery, after-effects, long-term expectations of recovery, any further treatment.	Patient can explain purpose and effects of surgery and long-term outcome.
(2) *Two days prior to discharge*	
i. Discuss journey home. Put on outdoor clothes, pad wound. ii. Anticipate experience of first week at home. Convince patient he should control his recovery. Advise on rests and walks and fatigue.	Patient and family have plans for journey, are aware of fatigue and importance of gradually increasing exercise.
iii. Explain any drugs to be taken. Advise on diet.	They can name any drugs and understand their purpose and administration.
(3) *One day prior to discharge*	
i. Long-term goals repeated. Patient is the best judge of how much to do. Improves positive health objectives. ii. Discuss activities important to patient, driving, employment, golf, sex, etc. iii. Give means of contacting staff if required and indicate it is welcomed.	Appears confident of what he will do, or try in the next few weeks. Has written suggestions and reminders.
(4) *Day of discharge*	
i. Dressed with extra protection for wound. ii. Supplied with medication, has repeated when this is to be taken. iii. Has out-patient appointment and ward telephone number and Nurse M's name. iv. Patient is reminded of optimistic aims, and that he controls his own pace!	Discharged with three days' preparation, a good understanding, a written plan and positive outlook!

A possible plan for a patient with major abdominal surgery is provided in Table 6.

A brief account of relevant aspects to include in teaching will now be given. The most important aspect which Lineham (1966) found to be raised by patients was 'how much they should do at home'. Most evidence suggests that progressive exercise daily should be continued as long as this is asymptomatic. They should be encouraged to do a little more each day without causing undue fatigue. If they feel breathless or pain they should rest for a while and resume later. However, they should be warned that they will feel fatigued and they will therefore need to make a positive effort to be active. To recondition their muscles, walking is said to be most beneficial (Preston, 1977), possibly accompanied for the first few times outside.

Other activities should also be graduated. Sexual intercourse can sometimes be slightly uncomfortable post-operatively; it may be easier in a side-to-side position. This is also recommended for post coronary thrombosis patients by Croog *et al.* (1968). As patients are sometimes reluctant to ask [Lineham (1966) showed this], staff on the ward, possibly a member of the same sex, should introduce this part of the teaching plan.

Lifting and bending often concerns patients, in particular those who have abdominal surgery, such as herniorrhapy or hysterectomy. Although the evidence is incomplete, it is, once more, the patients who are most able to decide when they feel comfortable and are able to bend and lift. Advice should be tailored to the individual's capability, but all patients should be taught how to lift to avoid strain. The stronger the muscles were previously, the more rapidly they recover. Johnston (1978) showed that female patients often found cleaning the bath and hoovering, which involved lifting and stretching, were the last domestic chores to be resumed.

In principle, it should be the patient who controls how rapidly he resumes his normal healthy activities. This should be clearly understood by the patient, who then knows that there is no 'typical' or 'correct' speed or pattern for his recovery progress. However, some staff (and patients) feel that more specific guidelines are necessary and have produced a written sheet of instructions. Although these can be individually tailored to some extent (by altering the lengths of time for certain activities), they tend to be brief and only cover the most general topics, like driving, returning to work, marital relations and symptoms which necessitate contacting the doctor. They can, of course, be used as a focus for further conversation about recovery at home with the patient and his family.

Pains in the wound, in the back and limbs may also prevent much activity for convalescent surgical patients. Stiffness is also a consequence of a passive hospitalization. Apart from using their supply of paracetamol or aspirin, patients may benefit from massage, warm baths or swimming. Wound pain may persist or be intermittent. Nerve regrowth or catgut sutures delayed in dissolving can cause sharp pain. This usually resolves in a few weeks, although a persistent problem may mean further medical treatment.

Patients' dietary needs should always be discussed well before hospital discharge. Although individual needs differ, it is wise to eat smaller meals than usual, at first to avoid indigestion which can give rise to intense discomfort. Peristalsis tends to be sluggish and constipation can present a problem in the early stages of recovery. As patients tolerate more exercise this problem subsides.

Adhering to medications and advice is an obviously important part of recovery. Evidence that non-compliance is so frequent (Marston, 1970) indicates that this vital aspect of recovery should be represented in any discharge teaching. Ley and Spelman's (1967) code of practice is useful. Simple explanations and notes of what drugs are for, what will happen if they are discontinued prematurely, and when they should be taken are fundamental. But others (Blackwell, 1976; Matthews, 1975) have shown that it may be helpful for drugs to be taken as part of the daily routine with a regular activity which becomes a reminder. When staff consider how this may be done with the patient and then rehearse this during the days prior to discharge, this may start to create a habit. When several long-standing prescriptions are required, patients may like to keep a drug diary. Omissions can then be identified and difficulties discussed on return visits. This may seem over-complicated but prescriptions should only be made if they are essentially beneficial and really need to be taken.

If the patient's family, or spouse in particular, seems unduly worried about the recovery process, further counselling may be needed. As Mayou *et al.* (1978) found, it may well be the wife who is over-anxious and protective and prevents complete confidence or optimal activity levels for the patient. It sometimes helps to have a separate session with them just to hear their view of the patient's illness, treatment and recovery and to reassure them that it is safe, and indeed beneficial, for the patient to do as much as he can without feeling tired. Sexual intercourse may not be of chief concern at the time of discharge, but it would be appropriately discussed during this session.

This type of information may appear so obvious to doctors, nurses or physiotherapists, but the majority of follow-up studies demonstrate that patients frequently want such guidance and, what is more, do not seem able to ask for this (Lineham, 1976). In the days prior to discharge, nurses in particular should facilitate opportunities for focussed discussion to allow for such questions as well as planning how and when to present all the information they consider the patient may need.

Coordination and continuity of care after hospital discharge

A friendly and open atmosphere on a ward, which encourages patients' questions and comments may be the best way of ensuring that patients feel able to contact staff, if needed, when they return home. However, Skeet (1970) found that, despite patients' rcports of friendship from staff, there were great problems due to inadequate planning for discharge and subsequent levels of community care. Her findings were not dissimilar to those of the Royal Commission (1979) when 12% of patients had less than 24 hours' warning of their discharge and subsequent difficulties with travel arrangements and liaison with GPs.

Skeet's recommendations are therefore still relevant to our present situation. As she said, communication between hospital and district care could always be improved, but some simple direct means of contact should be considered more frequently. Telephone calls from hospital doctors or ward sisters to GPs or the patient's own professional helpers are quicker and cheaper than letters which can follow later. Nurses should perhaps be particularly careful to encourage friendship or neighbour support when discharging someone who lives alone, even if they appear mobile on discharge. Simpson and Levitt's (1981) work also provides insights into special needs for discharge care, and highlights how variable social and health care can be, even in the UK, where such provisions are statutory requirements. As Hockey (1968) found, supporting services often did most to support the relatives, even with chronically ill dependents.

In many studies (Hockey, 1968; Roberts, 1975; Skeet, 1970; Ferguson, 1961), it was domestic (home) help, help with shopping and company which patients most needed. Specific nursing care procedures were carried out but reassurance and information were still required by a large proportion of patients upon returning home. Voluntary services were found to be most useful, yet Skeet and more recently a study by Gay and Pitkeathley, (1979) showed that they could do more if staff would request this. Such help as car driving, and warming and re-stocking an empty house ready for the patient's return, and paying regular visits in the early stages of recovery for those who lack company was offered and appreciated, yet underused. Perhaps staff underestimate the benefit of this type of help which others have relied on for so long.

It is perhaps not always sufficient to ensure that communications are rapid—they must be relevant. With more and more specialist treatment, GPs and district nurses require more information on care and recovery objectives. Otherwise they may dissuade a vigorous approach to return to health activities, as Mayou *et al.* (1978) and Wilson-Barnett (1981) found. When difficult procedures are necessary at home, nurses may welcome a word with ward staff on how this was managed. The trend for specialist teams, such as renal, diabetic and terminal care teams, to make home visits may help patients, but their skills and goals should be shared with general district staff. If the hospital is seen as part of the community, as Kratz (1976) and many others suggest, there may be much less conflict over continuous care.

New plans to solve the hospital–home gap, such as the liaison sister, are certainly becoming more evident. Sisters who nurse or get to know patients while they are in hospital and then care for them afterwards, seem to be accepted and helpful to patient, family and other staff. Few such posts have been systematically evaluated, but Jones and Hadley (1980) found that for terminal patients this enabled more patients to return home as they wished, and gave tremendous support to the family at such a time of need (Hockey, 1968).

For the general patient who returns for one or two out-patient visits and has not been seen to be in need of scarce community resources, nurses in particular could do more during this return visit to the hospital. Although clinics are busy, there are opportunities for supportive teaching and research. Nurses and doctors need to appreciate the importance of this visit to the patient who, after all, has missed work or cancelled other meetings to attend. Patients are usually seeking the doctor's advice or decision and often wait a long time for this, as the Royal Commission (1979) showed. From the patients' point of view they need to be able to ask questions, remember the answers and understand what has been said. Ley and Spelman (1967) showed how incomplete their recall and comprehension was and concluded that this must be a major reason for non-compliance. These aspects suggest a major role for the nurse. There is no justification for nurses in clinics to act as receptionists.

Many of these ideas have already been aired (Wilson-Barnett, 1981), and in principle involve nurses interviewing patients to assess their purpose for the consultation, answering any questions they might have where possible and recording their experiences since hospitalization or their last visit. They may well advise patients to write down any questions for the doctor or, if they seem diffident, to accompany them when seeing the doctor.

Reporting on patients' recovery experiences should be done systematically but the pressure of time during out-patient consultations frequently prevents this. Unless there is an accurate assessment of problems, recovery rates and risk factors, practice cannot be scientific. Preston (1977) strongly recommends a standard completion form for out-patient use. This may well resemble that suggested for post-operative coronary artery bypass graft patients in Chapter 5. With these data, which obviously have to be analysed and understood, staff would be armed with ways of identifying high-risk patients, information to prepare future patients, researched evidence comparing the outcome of their work and, hopefully, a greater sense of purpose in out-patient work.

Concluding Remarks

This book has been devoted to convincing medical and health-care staff that there are definite indications for improving the results of acute care. These point to better management in hospital, preparation for discharge and continuity of care and require more awareness that patients have needs, often unexpressed, for guidance during their recovery. Emphasis on acute care and technology has advanced medical knowledge and benefited patients, but it is no longer good professional practice to leave it to the generalist doctor or nurse in the community to pick up the patient (pieces) in the early stages of recovery without more assistance. Our practice should be orientated to preventing further complications, unnecessary psychological morbidity and incomplete recovery. It should be aimed at optimal levels of health, involving the patient in his own treatment and health training and towards promoting research by being honest over inadequacies in knowledge.

References

Blackwell, B. (1976). Treatment adherence. *British Journal of Psychiatry,* **129**, 513–531.

Bourke, J. B., Lear, P. A., and Taylor, M. (1981). Effects of early return to work after elective repair of inguinal herniorrhaphy. Clinical and financial consequences at one year and three years. *Lancet*, **ii**, 623–625.

Croog, S., Levine, S., and Lurie, Z. (1968). The heart patient and the recovery process. A review of the directions of research on social and psychological factors. *Social Science and Medicine,* **2**, 111–164.

Ferguson, T. (1961). Aftercare of the hospitalised Patient. *British Medical Journal,* **i**, 1242–1244.

Gay, P., and Pitkeathley, J. (1979). *When I Went Home . . . A Study of Patients Discharged from Hospital.* King Edward's Fund for London.

Griffiths, M., Waters, W. E., and Acheson, E. D. (1979). Variation in hospital stay after inguinal herniorrhaphy. *British Medical Journal,* **i**, 787–789.

Hockey, L. (1968). *Care in the Balance.* Queen's Institute of District Nursing, London.

Johnson, J. E., Dobbs, J. M., and Leventhal, H. (1970). Psychosocial factors in the welfare of surgical patients. *Nursing Research,* **19**, 18–29.

Johnston, M. (1978). Assessing recovery from surgery. *Paper presented at British Psychological Society Annual Conference,* York.

Jones, D., and Hadley, A. (1980). Evaluation of a clinical nurse specialist post. *Internal Report.* The Brompton Hospital, London.

Kratz, C. R. (1976). Some determinants of care of patients with stroke who were nursed in their own houses. *Journal of Advanced Nursing,* **1**, 89–96.

Ley, P., and Spelman, M. (1967). *Communicating With the Patient.* Staples Press, St. Albans.

Lineham, D. T. (1966). What does the patient want to know? *American Journal of Nursing,* **66**, 1066–1070.

Marston, M. V. (1970). Compliance with medical regimens: a review of the literature. *Nursing Research,* **19**, 313–332.

Matthews, D. (1975). The non-compliant patient. *Primary Care,* **2**, 284–294.

Mayou, R., Foster, A., and Williamson, B. (1978). Psychosocial adjustment in patients one year after myocardial infarction. *Journal of Psychosomatic Research,* **22**, 447–453.

Preston, T. A. (1977). *Coronary Artery Surgery: A Critical Review.* Raven Press, New York.

Raffle, A. (1976). *Medical Aspects of Fitness to Drive. A Guide for Medical Practitioners.* Medical Commission on Accident Prevention, London.

Redman, B. K. (1975). *The Process of Patient Teaching in Nursing.* Third edition. Mosby, New York.

Roberts, I. (1975). *Discharged from Hospital.* Royal College of Nursing, London.

Royal Commission on the National Health Service (1979). *Patients' Attitudes to the Hospital Service.* Research Paper 5. H.M.S.O., London.

Simpson, P. J. G., and Levitt, R. (1981). *Going Home.* Churchill-Livingstone, Edinburgh.

Simpson, J. E. P., Cox, A. G., Meade, T. W., Brennan, P. J., and Lee, J. A. (1977). 'Right' stay in hospital after surgery: randomised controlled trial. *British Medical Journal,* **ii**, 1514–1516.

Skeet, M. (1970). *Home from Hospital.* The Dan Mason Research Committee, London.

Strasser, A. L. (1977). When should the heart patient go back to work? *Occupational Health and Safety,* **46**, i, 30–31.

Wilson-Barnett, J. (1981). Patients first! *Nursing Mirror,* **153**, 5, 21–22.

Index